Dolæus up

the gout b

To which is prefixed, an essay upon diet

Johannes Dolæus,

William Stephens

Alpha Editions

This edition published in 2021

ISBN : 9789355112651

Design and Setting By
Alpha Editions
www.alphaedis.com
Email - info@alphaedis.com

PREFACE.

Some Gentlemen of very great Worth, whose Desires I could not resist, engaged me in the Translation of the following Treatise of Dolaeus; *they thought it might be of Use to Persons afflicted with the Gout, to have an easier Way of coming at the Facts contained therein, by naturalizing it into our Language; to which I can only add my good Wishes, as I have done my Endeavours in this Publication; for its Usefulness must be judged of by the Event.*

In Examining Dolaeus *his Work, Many Things occurred to me not so agreeable to my Way of thinking about these Matters, as I could have wished consistent with my publishing thereof, without taking Notice of them; some necessary Things I apprehended to be omitted, some Appearances very odly accounted for, some Directions and Medicines too loosely and too generally recommended; and indeed, through the whole, too little Care taken of nicely distinguishing Constitutions and Habits, to which Directions of this Kind should be specifically adapted, and never applied but upon the most skillful and mature Advice that can be had. The too much Encouragement that hath been given to valetudinary People, by publishing such loose and undetermined Directions, have made them think themselves judges of many Things of great Consequence to their Lives and Health, for which they are in no Sort qualified, and is generally attended with many great and often fatal Inconveniencies: And because they don't always find Relief by applying to Physicians, from such Mischiefs as their own Errors, and the Neglect of timely Advice have brought upon them, they are apt to conceive a bad Opinion both of the Profession and its Professors.*

The History of Cures, recited by Dolaeus, *I take to be the most valuable Part of his Book; the Appearances that happen therein, may, I think, be accounted for upon other and more philosophical Principles, than the Author hath adapted thereto; upon this, and the foregoing Accounts, I had determined to have added Notes at such particular Places as were proper for me to animadvert upon; but I found they swelled to too great a Bulk, and would have too much interrupted the Author in his own Way of telling his own Story; which occasioned the changing thereof into the Form they now appear in, of a preliminary Essay.*

The principal Hints in the Essay are taken from some loose Papers I have had long by me upon those Subjects; many of them were collected upwards of fifteen Years ago, when I was a very young Adventurer in Physick; so that I don't pretend to call them all my own, yet I have had long and frequent Occasion to see the Truth of them confirmed in many Instances, and the Pleasure to find them embraced and applied, by some of the greatest Masters of our Profession both at Home and Abroad. It is a great Loss to Observations of this Kind, that the Motions and Quantities of Matter are so far beyond our Senses, as to be incapable of being reduced to any certain Measures, which prevents that strict Mathematical Certainty we have arrived at in the Knowledge of the Properties of Motion in larger Bodies, more within the Compass of our Senses; the Gravitation of the heavenly Bodies, and of Bodies upon our Earth, to their respective Centres, have been reduced to certain Measure; and that there are mutual, attractive and repellent Powers, which act in certain Distances and Positions, annexed to the smallest Particles of Matter, as the immediate Cause of several natural Appearances, is highly resonable to believe; but whatever Boasts have been made by some of the modern Philosophers of accounting for those Appearances upon this Principle, they have amounted to no more than Evidences of its Existence; for the Laws of its Action are not yet sufficiently known for such Purposes as I have been speaking of; so that we must content ourselves with the History of Nature, in its Appearances, which under the same Circumstances will ever be the same, or at least as long as we shall have Occasion to observe them, let their Causes be what they will.

I have avoided the Quotation of Authors through the whole, as much as possible, because I have observed that whatever Appearance of honesty there may be in attributing to every Author the Hints he may have furnished, yet, a Multiplicity of Quotations is generally imputed rather to the Vanity of appearing Book learned, than any thing else, except to skreen Defects under greater Names, by the Publisher's not making himself by this Means accountable for what he says; the first I think I have disclaimed, by declining the Occasion, and the latter could be of no Use to me, because I hold myself accountable in this Publication only for the Truth of the Facts, and the Honesty of the Intention, which is to contribute what lies in my small Sphere to the good of Mankind, my Friends, and my Profession.

AN ESSAY UPON DIET,
Applied chiefly to the
GOUT.

All Birds, Beasts, and Fishes, Insects, Trees, and other Vegetables, with their several Parts, grow out of Water and Watry Tinctures and Salts; and by Putrefaction return again into Watry Substances.

All the Parts of Animals and Vegetables are composed of Substances volatile and fixed, fluid and solid, as appears by their Analysis; and so are Salts and Minerals, so far as Chymists have been hitherto able to examine their Composition.

Sir Isaac Newton's *Opt. p. 350, 360.*

It is very well known in the History of Physick, that very great Changes have been brought about in the human Body by the Force of Diet, especially in chronical Cases, where the Application of Medicines hath proved ineffectual. Chronical Distempers, as they are longer in coming to their Period, so they occasion a more universal bad Habit of Body; and where there is a pretty universal Depravation either of the Solids or Fluids of a human Body, or of both, it is not to be expected that sudden Changes can happen to Advantage: As the Progress is slow, and the Changes from a good to a bad State imperceptible, and by Degrees, the Changes to a good State must be so too. In acute Diseases indeed Medicines are more immediately necessary, because the Changes being quick and violent, immediate and sometimes violent Remedies become necessary; there being no Time to wait the slow and ordinary, tho' more certain, Methods of Change by the Alimentary Powers.

The Gout, of all chronical Distempers, requires least the Application of violent or uncertain Remedies: Tho' its pain be very intense, it comes very slow to its Period: Generally it is many Years, or the imprudent Application of Medicines, that brings it into the noble Parts, so as to endanger Life; purging by the Bowels hath frequently brought it into the Stomach; external Applications of repellent Plaisters have drove it into the Head; Applications of Mercurial Plaisters have brought on Paralytick Disorders: As we are not certainly acquainted with the particular Nature of the Gouty Matter, it is uncertain how to apply. That there is somewhat in the Part, not natural to the Body, which occasions the Pain, we know; what it is particularly we know not; the common Method of Nature is to evacuate it by the Pores of the Skin at certain Seasons, which requires the Part to be kept warm, and to attend upon the Operations of Nature for Relief; this, and the Uncertainty of Medicinal Applications, have brought *Patience and Flannel* to be Proverbial to the Gout.

Since the Cure of the Gout doth not with Safety admit the Application of sudden or violent Remedies, nor the Nature thereof require them; Physicians have, with very great Prudence, turned their Thoughts to other Methods of Cure; for this End, it was very proper to consider the Gout as the Distemper of the Rich and the Lazy, that it flows chiefly from Idleness and Fulness of Bread; that Persons afflicted therewith have naturally keen Appetites, and are apt to indulge in larger Quantities and cruder Kinds of Food, than the digestive Powers are able to deal with; that it chiefly happens to sedentary People; that upon the Approach of a Fit of the Gout, and during the Paroxysm, there are evident Marks of Indigestion in the Stomach and Bowels. If we add hereto the actual Relief that many Persons have found in the Use of a proper Diet, we shall not be at a Loss for a Reason, why Physicians should expect to find a more certain and easy Method of Cure in the Gout by Diet, than by any other Means.

It is not my Design at present to enter into the particular History of the Gout; this is very well known, and so accurately described by Dr. *Sydenham*, that it is needless; nor to enter into any long Detail of the History of the Alimentary Powers; this is likewise sufficiently known; nor to raise any Altercations about the particular Quality of the Gouty Matter, which is unknown, neither would the Knowledge thereof be much to my present Purpose. It will suffice to examine with Accuracy the Nature of Animal and Vegetable Diet, and the Habits they produce in the human Body, and to apply this to the Nature and Symptoms of the Gout.

The Knowledge of the particular Quality of the Gouty Matter is not absolutely necessary to our present Purpose; it is sufficient if it be made to appear, that the whole Habit of the Body may be changed by Diet. An Animal is entirely composed of the Food it is nourished by, the first *Stamen*, or Principle of Life, is most exceedingly small; and all that it afterwards receives its Growth from, may properly enough be called its Food: In oviparous Animals, and the same happens in viviparous ones, (tho' it be not so much within the Compass of our Observation) the first Nourishment is the White of the Egg, a Fluid very analogous to the *Serum* of the Blood, and the Subject of the Encrease is originally so small as almost to escape the strictest Enquiry.

Many, if not most Authors, who have entered into the particular Quality of the Gouty Matter, have placed it in an acrimonious acid Salt, and upon that Scheme have gone into the Method of a Milk and Vegetable Diet for the Cure. The Cure upon this Scheme seems to me not very rational, because Milk and Vegetables in their natural State tend to Acidity; and the

Chalky Substance of the Gout and Stone in the Bladder (which are pretty near akin) are soluble only by *Aqua fortis*, which is the strongest Acid. The Digestion of Animal Food, which is found to encourage, if not occasion the Gout, naturally tends to Alcalescence; and therefore there is more Reason to conclude the Gouty Matter to be Alkaline than Acid; but the Truth is, there are no evident Marks of either Acid or Alkali in the Animal Juices of an healthy Body, nor of any other Salt but Sea Salt, which is taken in with the Food, and as it is incapable of Change, passes thro' the Vessels of the Body. There is indeed an Acidity discoverable in the Bowels and lacteal Vessels, which is doubtless owing to the acid Food, for it doth not change its Nature, till it be thoroughly assimilated with the Blood in several Circulations; for even in the Chyle an Acid is sometimes discoverable: This Acid is lost in the Milk, which is but one Change farther, tho' even in this it is evident there is some Tendency that Way, because of its Disposition to turn sowre by standing. As there is doubtless Air in the Blood, there must be somewhat Nitrous, because there is no Air without Nitre, and Nitre is an Acid, but cannot come within Imagination of occasioning the Gout. That the Gout should consist in an Acid, and be curable by acessent Aliment, the Gouty Chalk dissolved only by Acids, and the Aliment that occasions it alkalescent, would be very strange. On the contrary, there is as strong Evidence that the Gouty Matter is not perfect Alkali, neither is there any such Thing in the Juices of an healthy Body; for tho' Animal Juices naturally tend to Alkalescence, they putrify before they arrive at that State, so as to be incapable of Circulation: The Disposition of Animal Juices this Way is so strong, that if they were not continually diluted by fresh Portions of Chyle, they would arrive at that putrescent Alkaline State that would destroy the Animal, as is evident in the Case of Animals starved to Death. Twenty Days Fasting will not diminish the Quantity of the Blood so much as a large Bleeding, and in some Kinds of Consumptions the Diminution of the Solids and Fluids is much greater than could happen by being starved; but in the Case before us, the Juices turning Alkaline and Corrosive affect the tender Fibres of the Brain, and the Animal dies feverish and delirious: On the contrary, People have lived above twenty four Days upon Water only, which can happen no otherwise than by diluting the Fluids, and consequently keeping them from this Alkaline State. In short, if the Juices of an Animal Body were either Acid or Alkaline, so as to cause an Ebullition by Mixture of their Opposites, they would burst the Vessels.

I shall consider Vegetable Substances with regard to Diet, in the first Place, because they are the Original Food of all Animals, who either immediately are nourished thereby, or else feed upon such Animals as are nourished by them.

Vegetables receive their Food from the Air and Earth, by means of several Recipient Vessels placed in the Root and Bark, (analogous to the Lacteals in Animals) conveyed and diluted by a sufficient Quantity of Water: This Food thus received, which I shall beg Leave to call Vegetable Chyle, is digested and assimilated in the Course of Circulation, through the Vessels of the Plant, till it is converted into Vegetable Substance, and is formed into the several differing Vegetable Juices, Gums, and Resins, that are peculiar to each Species of Plants. The Remainder, after the proper Separations, is evaporated thro' the Pores of the Skin and through the Leaves, in the Manner of Animal Transpiration. I content myself here with this short Hint of Vegetable Nutrition, because I have treated it more at large and expresly in another Place: It is more material at present to examine the several Juices which circulate in the Vessels of Vegetables, because, in regard to Diet, they will appear to be the Matter of Animal Nutrition; for the Vessels of Plants are no other than meer Earth bound or connected together with Oyl, by the Means of some very powerful Attraction: This Earth is undissoluble by the utmost Force of Fire, since after burning a Plant in the open Fire, we find it left entire.

The Chyle of Plants seems to be made up of whatever Parts in the Earth are soluble in Water, so as to be capable of being received into the Absorbent or Recipient Vessels of Plants, before taken Notice of; and consequently may consist of Salts, Oyls, Fumes of Minerals, Metals, and other fossil Bodies, the putrified Parts of Animals and Vegetables. In its first State it is, to be sure, very crude; but by the Structure and Fabrick of the Plant, and the various Vessels it is strained thro', it is changed, elaborated, secreted, and assimilated into the Substance of the Plant; whence it follows, that in Vegetables are contained Salts, Oyl, Water, and Earth, and probably Metals too, for the Ashes of Vegetables yield somewhat which the Load-Stone attracts.

This Juice, when it first enters the Root, is Earthy, Watry, Poor, and Acid, it is in the Form of a fine and subtle Water; the nearer it is to the Root, the more it retains of its proper Nature, the further it is from the Root, and the more Action it hath sustained it approaches nearer to a Vegetable Nature, as will appear by pursuing it a little further. In the Trunk and Branches it is further prepared, tho' even here it is Watry and Acid, as appears by tapping Trees at the proper Season: It is more concocted in the Bud, where the Leaves coming to be unfolded, serve as Lungs for the further Preparation of it in the Course of Circulation; in the Flower, Leaves and Parts of Generation, it is still further elaborated, and becomes in its utmost Perfection, fine enough to preserve and nourish the Embryo in the Seeds of Plants. This Nutritious Juice or Chyle is pretty universal, and is found in every Part of a Plant, but more or less in Quantity, and more or less impregnated with the more Elaborate Juices, according to the Number and Degree of its Circulations. It seems to be the universal Diluent and Conveyer of other and more elaborated Particles. Besides what I have mentioned, there are Juices particular to particular Parts of Plants; as Oyl, Wax, and Manna to the Leaves; Volatile Oyl or Spirit, and Honey to the Flower; a very fine Essential Oyl or Balm to the Seed, and that in great Quantity; Oyl, Balm, Pitch, Resin and Gum to the Bark: Besides which, there is a Juice peculiar to each Plant, and received in Vessels of its own, in which a good Deal of its Specifick Nature may consist, (for it is not reducible to any of those before mentioned) most of the *English* Authors call this the proper Juice of the Plant, but *Boerhave* and later Writers call it the Blood. I should digress too much to enter into the natural History of these several Parts of Vegetables; my Design at present reaching no further than with Respect to their Assimilation into Animal Substance; and therefore I refer to the Authors who have expresly treated of these Matters, and proceed to examine Vegetable Juices in another Light.

The Juices of Plants are Watry, Saline, Oily, Spirituous, Gummy, Balsamick, or Resinous, all discoverable by Art. The Water is generally found in the Absorbent Vessels of Plants, but mixed with a Proportion of Salt, which, tho' always soluble in Water, otherwise appears of very different Nature in different Plants, and differs in Degree of Volatility.

The Oily Part is that which grows Fluid at the Fire, proves inflammable, and will not unite with Water, without the Intervention of Salt. It is seldom obtained pure from Vegetables, because therein it exerts so very strong an attractive Force upon Salt, Water, and Earth, that nothing less than the Force of Fire, assisted by the Action of the Air, can separate them, as appears in *Helmont's* Everlasting Coal.

The Spirituous Parts of Plants, or those which contain the Odour and Taste, are very volatile, will mix with Water, and sometimes burn in the Fire, the Oyl of the Vegetable being here greatly attenuated, broke, and subtilized; as appears by its being exhalable by the Heat of the Summer Sun, so as to form the particular Atmosphere of the Plant, and fill the Air with Particles that affect our Senses even at some Distance.

Gums are such Productions of Vegetables, as will mix with Water, dissolve over the Fire, and burn away, being tough viscid Substances, and contain a large Proportion of the Oyl and Salt of the Plant. Balsams are native Oyl of Vegetables, brought to a thick Consistence, but containing a large Proportion of an acid Spirit and Salt: However, they differ greatly from the Oyls they afford. Lastly, Resins are such Productions of Vegetables, as being hard and dry, prove brittle in the Cold, soluble by Heat, inflammable and misceable with Oyl, but not with Water.

It would be endless to give an Account of the particular Qualities of the proper Juices of Plants; since these differ in different Plants, and many Times in different Parts of the same Plant. There is a much greater Variety in Vegetable than in Animal Nature; and a much greater Difference in the Juices of one than of the other; for the Number of different Plants known and used very much exceeds the Number of different Animals known and used; and particular Plants have greater Variety of Juices than particular Animals; whose Juices (if I may so speak) are more homogenial than those of Plants. This will appear more evidently by comparing what hath been here said, with the Consideration of Animal Substances with Regard to Diet.

I have hitherto considered Vegetables in their natural State, but before we can apply what hath been laid down to Animal Diet, we must consider some Changes many of them undergo, before they are used. The Chief of these happens by Fermentation, the Effects of which upon Vegetables deserve to be considered; since Bread, Wine, and Malt Liquors, so great a Part of our common Food, are prepared from Vegetables that have gone thro' this Operation, or are mixed with Ferments in their Preparation.

Fermentation is a Change in Vegetables by Means of some intestine Motion, the Effect whereof is, that in Distillation there arises a volatile inflammable Liquor, capable of mixing with Water, commonly called Spirits; or if the Fermentation be so managed as to produce Vinegar, thence arises in Distillation a watry, thin, acid Liquor, capable of extinguishing Fire. I have here only mentioned the Effects of Fermentation; what this intestine Motion is, or its Cause, I do not pretend to describe, because I do not know it: Its Effects are very well known to be either a vinous or an acetous Liquor, and they are producible from all Vegetables, and from Vegetables only; for all the Art yet known will never gain such Spirits either from Fossils or Animals: Putrefaction, Digestion, and Effervescence are all done by intestine Motions, but will neither produce Wine nor Vinegar; so that in this Light Fermentation is confined to Vegetables.

It needs no very deep Enquiry into the History of Fermentation, to know, that in Wine (by which Name I understand all fermented Vegetable Liquor, Ale, Beer, Mead, and all artificial Wines, as well as that made from the Grape) the Spirituous Parts of the Vegetable are so volatilized and loosened, that very small Heat raises them from the other Parts of the Liquor, even many fly off upon being exposed to the Air: The viscid, oily, and glutinous Parts of Vegetables are so broke and separated, and the Spheres of their mutual Attractions so diversified, that they are no longer retained. Before Fermentation, the longer you boil the Decoction of any Vegetable, its oily and spirituous Parts are more concentrated, and little besides Water, and some essential Oyl goes away; after Fermentation the

Spirit goes away, and the Water remains: This is commonly known to Brewers and Distillers.

What is next observable in this Change is, that the essential Salt is thrown from the Body of the Liquor thus fermented, and adheres to the Side of the Vessel wherein the Liquor is deposited, and crystallizes into Tartar. In Vinegar this Salt is kept in the Mass of the Fluid (the Oyl being thrown off) where uniting with the aqueous and spirituous Parts, it turns sowre, and becomes Vinegar by Means of that Fermentation. After this no Tartar can be generated from it, nor any inflammable Spirit obtained; but on the contrary, a watry, poor, acid Liquor, capable of extinguishing Fire, rises first from the Still. In Wine, the volatile Salt and Oyl of the Vegetable are attenuated and reduced into one Spirit; Vinegar is the essential Salt of Wine made more acid by a new Fermentation, and intimately mixed with the watry and spirituous Parts of the same.

The Spirit produced from the Distillation of Wine is a Liquor of such active Parts, and capable of effecting such Changes in animal Bodies, that it ought to be retained entirely to Medicine; but since it is too much used in Diet, it may be proper to remember it under that Head.

I must take Notice of one other Change in Vegetables, and that is what they undergo by Putrefaction, because it Approaches somewhat to animal Digestion, and gives us some Sort of Notion of the Manner of converting vegetable into animal Substances.

It is very well known, that if a Quantity of green recent Vegetables be heaped up together, and pressed down, they will in a little Time begin to heat in the Middle, and in the Course of eight or ten Days will have passed by Degrees to a violent Heat, so as sometimes to flame and burn away; this Mass acquires a putrid, cadaverous, feculent Taste and Smell, and turns into a soft, pappy Substance, resembling human Excrement in Scent, and putrified Flesh in Taste; and by all the Tryals that can be made, gives us no mark of vegetable Substance, but is entirely turned into an animal one: For upon Distillation it yields a Water of an urinous Scent; a white, volatile, dry, alkaline Salt; a volatile, alkaline, oily Salt; and a thick fetid Oyl, all the same that are producible from animal Substances; and lastly, (which is the nicest Criterion between vegetable and animal Substances) if the Remainder be calcined in an open Fire, it will not yield the least Particle of fixed Salt, which all Vegetables whatsoever are known to do.

All Vegetables whatever are subject to this Putrefaction (and indeed Animals too) and all specifick Differences are destroyed by it: It is evidently caused by Fire itself collected or included within the subject; and seems to be a general Law of Nature, wisely established, to produce wonderful Changes in the World, and to prevent the Indolence of Matter; this active

Principle or Medium giving an easy and reciprocal Transition of vegetable into animal Substances, and of animal into vegetable. I think it cannot be out of the Way here to observe, that the Change which the Aliment suffers in the human Body, is in some Measure reducible to this; for if a Man should live entirely upon acid Vegetables, acid Bread, and Fruits, drink Rhenish Wine, no Part of his Body or Juices would, upon Distillation, or other Tryal, yield the least Portion of an acid or fixed Salt, but constantly a volatile Alkali. There cannot indeed be supposed any perfect Putrefaction in the Bodies of Animals; for so soon as any Thing contained therein tends this Way, it is discharged as Excrement; all the Acids of the Aliment are subdued by the vital Powers of Animals, and converted into volatile Salts of an alkaline Nature; without an actual or real Putrefaction, yet by an Operation nearly approaching thereto: If these Salts were not discharged, before Putrefaction (as by examining the Excrement it appears they are) they must produce such terrible Effects as would immediately destroy the Animal.

In examining vegetable Substances as Food, we must consider them as eaten Raw, as prepared by the Arts of Cookery, and as subjected to Fermentation. In the first Case they are sometimes the Food of Men, always of Animals that we feed upon; in the others the Food of Men alone.

Raw Vegetables that become Parts of Animals, are bruised, ground, and comminuted by the proper animal Organs, and mixed with animal Juices in their Passage. By this Means their Juices are expressed; such of them as are capable of mixing with Water naturally, or by the intermediate Assistance of the Bile, are formed into one common fluid Mass or Chyle, which constitutes the first Nourishment of Animals; whence the Blood, Serum, Lymph, and other animal Juices are formed. From what was said before, this appears to be the Water, impregnated with the essential Salt, the Spirit, some Portion of its essential Oyls, mixed with the Water by Means of the Salt and the Bile; these by the vital Powers are formed into a white Liquor, which is the Chyle, not unfitly represented in the common making of Emulsions from oily Seeds. The Chyle still retains its vegetable Nature, and somewhat specifick to the Vegetable it came from; but when it hath been circulated several Times thro' the Body, and thoroughly mixed with the Juices thereof, it acquires animal Properties; vegetable and animal Juices are pretty near of the same specifick Gravity, and consequently fit to repair each other; the different Impulses of Heat and Motion, with due Mixture, create the Difference; though this will always hold true, that an animal Body constantly repaired from vegetable Juices, cannot have so strong a tendency to a putrescent alkaline State, as a Body constantly repaired from animal Juices, already disposed to that State.

The common Effects of the Art of Cookery upon Vegetables, will be understood by what happens in the Decoction of Plants. In boiling any Plant, its most sublime fluid Part flies off, and indeed it is incapable of bearing a greater Heat than that of the Summer Sun, the Salts of the Plant are dissolved in the Water, and its thicker and grosser Oyl rises to the Top, like a fat Scum; so long as the Plant retains any Taste or Odour, change the Water as often as you please, there will constantly arise a fat, odorous, viscous, inflammable and frothy Matter, which can be no other than the Oyl of the Plant loosened from the Salts. In Proportion then, as the Salts are dissolved in the boiling Water, the Oyl attenuated, as it must be before it can be so far specifically lighter as to arise to the Top, we are to judge how far the Art of Cookery is serviceable in the Preparation of vegetable Diet.

From what was said before in relation to Fermentation, it is plain that the vegetable Oyls are much volatilized, rendred more active, and separated from the Salts; upon this Account it is, that they are endowed with an inebriating Quality, which is confined entirely to Wines, for no other Substance hath that Quality. No one was ever drunk with eating Grapes, or drinking Must or Wort before Fermentation. The stupifying Quality of Poppy, Henbane, Mandrakes, Nightshade, and other Plants of that Class, is very different from the Effects of Wine or its Spirit. The chief Effect of Fermentation, in Regard to Diet, is supposed to consist in rendring vegetable Substance less difficult to be overcome by the Action of animal Organs and Mixtures, and easier to the digestive Powers; but there are other good Effects not so commonly thought of; fermented vegetable Substance is very little subject to Putrefaction, and is a great Preservative against it. By the styptick Power that the Spirit is endowed with, the Tone of the Fibres is increased in Digestion, their Force enlarged, and consequently their Action greater upon the vegetable Parts, and a larger Quantity of animal Juices mixed with them; and it is no difficult Matter to imagine, that the inward Heat of an human Body should draw forth the Spirit of fermented Liquors.

The Parts of Vegetables most used in Food, are the Seeds of Plants, our common Bread and Drink being made from them: These, by what was said before, contain the most elaborated Juices, the greatest Quantity of fine Oyl and Spirit, and are consequently most fit for Nourishment; several Fruits are eaten Raw, because their Juices are concocted to the utmost Degree of Perfection, and contain, in greatest Quantity, the finest and most elaborated vegetable Oyl, mixed with the essential Salts peculiar to each, which would be lost in Decoction: But the coarser Parts of Vegetables, as Roots, Leaves, Stalks, unripe Fruits, and Flowers, require the Arts of Cookery to be exercised upon them, to render them more easily subject to the animal Powers, and assimilable to their Juices.

I design not to enter into the several specifick Differences of Vegetables, I hope I have said enough to explain their general Nature, and how they become reducible into animal Substances; I shall next consider these Substances in the same Manner.

By all the Tryals yet made upon animal Substances, they are resoluble into the same Parts with Vegetables, only differently modified; that is, as we saw before, Water, Earth, Salt and Oyl, the specifick Spirit being no other than Water impregnated with the specifick and highest rectified Oyl and Salt, the Water and Earth in both are individually the same; and though there be good Reason to imagine, that there is originally but one Oyl in Nature, and that the fixt Salt of Vegetables, and the volatile Salt of Animals, may be originally the same, since transmutable into one another; yet it is necessary to examine these two Principles in animal Substances, that by comparing them with what we before discovered in Vegetables, we may have some Notion of their Differences with Regard to their Use in Diet.

The great Excess of animal Heat and Motion, beyond what is necessary to Vegetables, the stronger and quicker Circulation of their Juices, necessarily require and occasion that the Oyls and Salts in animal Bodies should be differently modified from what they are in Vegetables. No Motion is performed in Animals without some Portion of Oyl, and perhaps Water too, to lubricate the Parts, and keep them supple; the Attrition would cause great Mischief, make the Motion uneasy, wear away and burn up the Parts, if they were not softned and moistned by an oily Fluid; and accordingly we find all the Muscles, Tendons, Joints and other Parts employ'd in Motion, to have Repositories of this Oyl placed about them, and that so artificially, that the Very Motion occasions the Diffusion of this Oyl upon them. There is an innate Principle of Heat or Fire, that attends the vital Powers, that may very well occasion the Change and Volatilization of Salts in animal Substances, in the same Manner as was before observed in the Putrefaction of Vegetables.

Animal Oyls differ according to the Principles inherent in them, for when freed from Earth and Salts (which is very difficult by Reason of their mutual Attractions under certain Circumstances) they appear to be simple and unactive, and the same in all animal Bodies.

By this Account then we are principally to regard the different Quantities and Degree of Volatility in these Salts, and the Degree of Consistence or Impregnation of animal Oyls with them. It must be observed, that the Salts in the Bodies of living Animals are not perfectly the same they appear to be, when extracted thence by chymical Resolutions; a great Alteration is made by the Fire, and a good deal by the Tendency all animal Substances have to Putrefaction, upon a Stagnation of their fluid Parts: Even in the Evaporation of human Blood (fresh drawn) by a gentle Fire, this Salt, though not perfectly fixed, will not rise, but only the Spirit: These Salts are of a mild attenuating Nature in healthy Bodies, whose vital Powers are sufficient to subdue the Substances they feed upon: But in such as have not that vital Power in that Degree, or commit Errors in Diet, where these Salts are not sufficiently attenuated, or the first Digestion stronger than the concoctive Powers or the Discharges, these Salts acquire Properties productive of many acute and chronical Diseases; (not within the Compass of this Enquiry) these may be prevented, and sometimes cured, by a strict Application to Diet, proper to correct the different Modifications of these Oyls and Salts.

I own it is pretty Difficult to determine the exact Degree of Volatility these Salts acquire in any particular Animal, or in different Parts of the same Animal; yet there are very evident Marks of a Defect, or Exceeding in the Volatility of these Salts, by examining the Discharges from Animals, by a greater or less Tendency to Putrefaction, by several Distempers more especially incident to human Bodies, and other Methods of Art to be met with in the History of Physick.

From what was said before, it is evident that an Animal, whose Juices are supplied from animal Juices, hath a more alkalescent Tendency than an Animal supplied with vegetable Juices; that is, the Salts are more highly volatilized, and impregnate the Oyls, Water, and other Fluids in a stronger Manner, and in greater Quantities; and in Fact, we find the Substance of such animal Bodies, as are fed upon Animals, or Use stronger Exercise, are more liable to Putrefaction, than the Substance of Animals that feed upon Vegetables, and are more slothful. Fish, Foxes, Hawks, Venison, Horses, have their Substance more liable to Putrefaction, and discover to our Senses more exalted Salts and Oyls, than tame Fowl, Sheep, and Oxen; the Juices of poisonous Animals have them still more exalted, as in the Viper.

Animal Substances being already assimilated, are more easily transmutable into other Animals, and therefore more nourishing than Vegetables; accordingly we find such Animals as are nourished by animal Food, to be more couragious, robust, active, bold, strong, than those which are nourished by Vegetables only. And even in Men, who have proper Organs for digesting both animal and vegetable Food, and consequently by Nature designed to use both, we find a remarkable Difference according to their Diet. The Inhabitants of fishing Towns, who may well be supposed to feed thereon, are strong, nervous and prolifick; and their Discharges, especially their Sweat, are often attended with a very strong rancid Smell. The Difference between these People, and some poor Peasants in the

Country, who have no other than vegetable Food, is too obvious to mention.

As to the Preparation of animal Diet, by the Arts of Cookery, for Use, it is needless to repeat what was before said under this Head in relation to Vegetables, the Manner being pretty much the same. I shall only just observe, that in boiling, the Salts and a good Portion of Oyl is dissolved, and attenuated in the Decoction, which makes the Decoction it self very nourishing; the animal Substance it self is much relaxed and softned, so that it may almost all be reduced to a Jelly or thick Oyl; by roasting, the Salts are more brought into Action, and the fluid Parts lessened; so that what remains is more highly impregnated therewith; in baking no Part evaporates, but both Salts and Oyls are loosened and exalted by the Heat in the Oven; these Differences are observable by the Taste, affect the digestive Powers in different Degrees, and are usefully attended to, in many different Habits of the human Body, too tedious now to be enumerated.

It is to be observed here (as before concerning Vegetables) that the nearer the nutritious Juices are to their Roots, the more they partake of the Nature of their Origine; but the more they are mixed with animal Juices, and the greater Number of animal Circulations they pass through, the more they acquire an animal Nature. The Chyle in Animals feeding upon Vegetables is Acid, and generally speaking it is so in Men, because their Diet is more so than otherwise. The Milk is less Acid than the Chyle, but turns perfectly so by standing. In the Blood this Tendency is lost, and the Salts from fixed become volatile. But there are Juices in animal Bodies, that have Salts of a much higher Degree of Volatility than the Blood, but when they arrive at too high a state of Alkalescence, they are discharged generally by Urine, or some other Excretion.

I do not here pretend to account for these Facts; that they are such is beyond Controversy, and I think it very agreeable to the Order of Nature, that they should depend upon some general Cause: If the Principle of Attraction be one, and from what Sir *Isaac Newton* hath delivered in his Opticks it bids very fair for it, though that great Philosopher was either too modest, or too knowing, to propose it as such, otherwise than by way of Quære; if the Principle of Attraction be an universal Cause in such Effects as we have been speaking of, may it not very justly be supposed, that when animal Decoctions turn sowre by standing, and so far put on a vegetable Nature, as to differ from the Course animal Substances take, when left to themselves, that the Salts are disunited, and put from the Sphere of one anothers mutual Attraction, so as perhaps to exert a repelling Power; and may not the same thing happen, when putrified animal Substance becomes Nourishment for vegetable Bodies, their Salts being disunited, and their mutual Attractions dissolved or overcome by the Attraction of Water,

Earth or other Parts, in the Substance which I before called vegetable Chyle? When Vegetables by Putrefaction acquire an animal Nature, are not the Salts brought into their Spheres of Attraction, so as to form different intestine Motions thereby, and to produce Heat, Fire, fetid Vapours, and Putrefaction?

Sir *Isaac Newton*, Opt. p. 362. compares a Particle of Salt to a Chaos, dense, hard, dry, and earthy in the Center; and rare, soft, moist and watry in the Circumference, and hence, says he, it seems to be that Salts are of a lasting Nature, being scarce destroyed unless by drawing away their watry Parts by Violence, or by letting them soak into the Pores of the central Earth, by a gentle Heat in Putrefaction, until the Earth be dissolved by the Water, and separated into smaller Particles, which by Reason of their smallness make the rotten Compound appear of a black Colour. Hence also it may be that the Parts of Animals and Vegetables preserve their several Forms, and assimilate their Nourishment; the soft and moist Nourishment easily changing its Texture by a gentle Heat and Motion, till it becomes like the dense, hard, dry, and durable Earth in the Center of each Particle. But when the Nourishment grows unfit to be assimilated, or the central Earth grows too feeble to assimilate it, the Motion ends in Confusion, Putrefaction and Death.

There is one animal Juice which deserves to be more particularly considered, not only because it is more used in our Food, than any other, but because it seems to partake of that just Medium between animal and vegetable Substances so desirable in our Diet, and that is Milk. It is neither Acid nor Alkaline; it seems to have enough of the animal Nature, to give strong and perfect Nourishment to animal Bodies, and to be easily assimilable to their Substance; enough of the Vegetable to prevent too strong a Tendency to a volatile Alkali; being a kind of Emulsion, or white, oily animal Liquor, prepared originally from Vegetables, and from which all the Parts of animal Bodies may receive their Nourishment and Growth. Many Persons have lived entirely upon Milk; and the Body of a Child may, at the End of some Months after its Birth, be considered as compounded of the Milk of its Nurse; the Parts it brought into the World being changed for others, supplied by the Nourishment.

Tho' Milk be of it self neither Acid nor Alkaline, it may not be amiss to take Notice of the Changes it undergoes upon being mixed with either, because hence we may determine its Agreement or Disagreement with different Constitutions. If Milk be mixed with Acids it coagulates into a Curd; if mixed with Alkalies, upon Heat it turns Yellow, then Red, and at length to a very deep dark Red, and by long continuance Black.

Milk taken from Animals that feed upon Vegetables, if suffered to stand in a clean glass Vessel, will of it self separate into two Parts; the lighter, and more oily, rising to the Top in the Form of Cream; both which in a few Days turn sowre, and at the End of ten or twelve Days, acquire a very considerable Degree of Acidity; but if the Animal it be taken from feed upon animal Diet, or have fasted too long, or be feverish, or use strong Exercise; it will in these Cases have a brackish or saline Taste, which is a strong Evidence of its Tendency to Putrefaction, and accordingly instead of turning sowre, it will turn rancid, and run into an Ichor.

It may fairly be concluded from hence, that Milk is not proper Food in acid Constitutions; for if Milk, upon the Mixture of Acids, turn into Curds and Whey, it is reasonable to expect, that if it be taken by Persons whose Bodies abound with Acids, it shall be separated into a thin serous Fluid, and a strong Coagulum; which turning grumous, may cause Obstructions in the *Viscera*, while it ceases to be mixed and diluted with the *Serum*, which instead of performing that Office, may go off in the Discharges of the Skin, or of Urine, leaving the Body pale, faint and weak; and hence may arise many chronical Distempers, foreign to our Purpose to enumerate.

The Change of Colour in Milk, by Alkalies, from White to Red, gives a very evident Reason for the easy Transmutation of the Chyle into Blood, when it leaves its vegetable Nature, and puts on an Animal one; and is a further Confirmation of the Doctrine hitherto laid down. The Appearances that are observable in the Changes Milk undergoes, when left to itself, instruct us in the Choice of such kind as is most proper for Nourishment; which is principally to be regarded, where the Animal is entirely fed with Milk, which is the Case of Children at the Breast; and what happens to Children, may with proper Allowances be applied to older Bodies. If a Nurse feed entirely upon Flesh Meats, Fish, and Broths, or be hot and feverish, or use much or violent Exercise, some of which often happen to be the Case in wealthy Families, the Milk grows Yellowish, and by standing will turn rancid, the Child manifests an Aversion to it, and becomes hot, red, and feverish; on the contrary, if the Nurses Food be too much enclined to Acidity, which is often the Case of poor People, the Child shall be subject to Flatulencies, preternatural Distention of the Body, and paleness of the Flesh: The Milk for Food ought to be perfectly white and clear, the Animal that gives it, not suffered to fast long before, and used for Food as soon as possible after it is milked; for thus it is had in its most perfect and natural State.

Before I leave the History of Diet, I cannot but take Notice, that as much Irregularity is committed in the Quantity, and Time of taking our Food, as in the Qualities or Properties thereof. From what hath been said it appears, that true Nutrition consists in the proper Assimilation of the Food to the Vegetable, or animal Body that takes it in; if the Powers of the Body be sufficient to assimilate what it takes in in a proper Manner, and to throw forth what it doth not need, or what is unfit for Assimilation, let the Food be what it will, the Body will be well nourished; on the contrary, if what be taken in be too strong to be changed by the digestive Powers, or the Powers of the Body too weak to expell it, that Body must be changed to a bad Habit; which, in its utmost Degree, is the Case of Plants and Animals that are poisoned. If the Body be oppressed with Loads of the most proper Food, more than the digestive Powers are able to deal with, or than there are animal juices sufficient to mix with for the proper Assimilation; those Powers must be weakened, the Fibres, being stretched beyond their Tone, lose of their Force, and what Foods are taken in, not being sufficiently acted upon by the Solids or Fluids of the Body, take the Course they would naturally have done out of the Body, and turn to Corruption, and Humour. When this happens to be the Case in human Bodies, upon a Stoppage of any of the great Discharges, as of Perspiration, by taking Cold, they become Subject to Fevers, and other acute Diseases, and Obstructions of the tender Bowels, chiefly the Liver and Lungs, which bring on several chronical Diseases, more especially the Dropsy and Asthma; for it is observable, that all overfed Animals have large Livers subject to Putrefaction, and are short winded.

I know no exact Way of determining the Quantities of our Food, and of the Changes inducible upon the Body, by the Quantities only, (before Pain and Sickness teach the Exceeding, when perhaps it may be past Remedy) but the Balance, and yet a Man would run the Hazard of being turned into Ridicule, that should gravely talk to People of weighing their Food or their Bodies, at certain Times. The cravings of Nature, and the returns of Appetite are thought to be better Indications for a supply, than the Weight of the Body, and so indeed they would be, if left to themselves; but we eat without Hunger, drink without Thirst, and lie a bed at times unnatural to sleep. I need not add that these are the People that want most the Helps of Medicine. The Quantities of Food, and the unnatural Encrease of the Body may be attended to, without running into ridiculous Extreams of nicety; and after the Rules are once settled, these things may be known without living in a Pair of Scales with *Sanctorius*. I can affirm it from certain Experience, that the keeping the Body to a certain standard of Weight, is a great preservative of Health; and many acute, and chronical Diseases may be foreseen, and prevented by it, and this is known by weighing once or twice a Month with less trouble than paring ones Nails, and regulating the Quantity of Food accordingly; so true is the Aphorism of *Sanctorius*, that if such Kinds, and such Quantities, be daily added to the Body as go off, and the Exceedings discharged, lost Health will be recovered, and present Health preserved.

Among the chronical Distempers, which owe their Origine to irregularities in Diet, the Gout is neither the least considerable nor frequent; though perhaps the best and least dangerous Way of clearing the Blood of the morbid Matter; for it naturally tends to the Extreams, and is generally so great a Tyrant, that it will suffer no other Distemper to rage but itself; upon this Account it is that People wish for, and are complimented upon the Gout, as an Indication of the vital Powers being in such Strength and Vigour, as to drive forth the gouty Matter; and it is no wonder that Persons should wish such active, fiery Particles, as the gouty Matter seems to consist of, fixed to a certain Joint, and expelled the Body, when they are floating through the Mass of Juices, and disorder the whole Machine, which is often the Case of gouty Persons before it fixes: The gouty Salts (if they be Salts, as most probably they are) appear to be active, sharp, pungent, fiery Principles, and when, by the Force and Heat of the Body, they are brought into Action, are not improperly termed concentrated Fire it self; and indeed the Effects of their Action manifest something not very different therefrom, by calcining the animal Substance into Chalk or Lime, or somewhat approaching thereto, in the Knots of gouty Joints: Their Volatility may Occasion their being more easily brought into a State of Action, but at the same Time makes their Expulsion out of the Body quicker and easier. A fit of the Gout is no other than an attempt of Nature to collect and expell these Salts out of the Body, which, if successfully performed, leaves the Person free from the Gout, till such Time as from the natural Course of the Food, or other Causes, the Blood and Juices become again overcharged with gouty Matter, to such Degree, that Nature attempts the same Way of Relief it before experienced, and occasions another Fit.

From this Account it appears, that if any thing be to be done during the Time of a Fit, which is the Season many Persons very preposterously attend a Cure, it can only be by supporting the Powers of the Body, to enable Nature, to go on with its Work: (For it must be considered, that the Symptoms of Pain arise from the Action of the Body in that Work, as well as from the Action of the gouty Salts;) and by promoting the natural Discharges from the Part affected, by gentle heat and Warmth; all external Applications, foreign to these Ends, are useless, and generally speaking dangerous. Indeed if any thing may safely be applied in this Case, for these Ends, some Preparation of the Poppy seems to me to be the most promising, and least hazardous. This Plant is endowed with Powers that soften and attenuate in a great Degree, gently promote and encrease the Motion of the Juices, and occasion in Bodies properly disposed, as great, if not greater Discharges by the Skin, than any other Medicine yet discovered. If we add to this its particular Property of easing Pain, may we not justly form great Expectations from it? Its Virtues given inwardly, in the Case we are speaking of, have been long known and experienced; its outward Application hath not, that I know of, been mentioned before; and I would be understood now rather to mention it, than recommend it. I have tried it in about half a Dozen Persons, the better half of which found immediate and wonderful Relief from it, and those who did not, found no inconvenience, to my thinking, chargeable upon the Medicine; though perhaps I am fond enough, like other Patrons of new Tryals, to impute the want of Success to other Causes, than to a Deficiency in the Medicine; I only mention the thing, not being thoroughly satisfied about it, for want of sufficient Tryal. But thus far I may venture to assert, that this, or any other external Applications, are neither to be unwarily or unskilfully ventured upon.

Some Authors of good Note have recommended purging the Bowels upon the Recess of the Gout, and during the Intervals of the Fit, as a proper preventive Cure in the Gout. That keeping the alimentary Passages clean, and in good Order, is of Use not only in the Gout, but in several other Distempers, is undoubtedly true; but how far this may be attended with a weakening of the Fibres of the Stomach, and how far the gouty Salts, already lodged in the Blood and Juices, may be drawn into these Parts, so as to act thereon, deserves very well to be considered. The Tendency of Nature is to drive the gouty Humour to the Extreams, and expell it forth of the Body; the Tendency of purging by the Bowels, further than cleansing the first Passages, is to draw the gouty Humour thither, and expell it by Siege. The Consonancy of these Tendencies may be seen without any Witchcraft; but a very accurate Judgment is necessary to distinguish at what Time, or in what Degree, the Juices of the Body are impregnated with the gouty Matter, so as to determine upon purging with Safety, or what Progress they have made in their Collection, and Tendency to the Joints, to venture to disturb Nature, in her own way of discharging them. Purging during the Time of a Fit is always avoided even by the Patrons of habitual gentle Purging out of it, and a Looseness is esteemed a very dangerous Symptom at that Time; sure I am from Experience, that many gouty Persons, who have run into the Practice of habitual Purging, even with those Medicines that are most strengthning, have found very bad Effects from that Custom, have been afterwards less able to withstand the Attacks of the Gout, have had more frequent and longer Returns, have at length sooner sunk under it, and fallen into worse Habits of Body, than others who have avoided that Practice: There may no doubt be a Necessity for the Use of evacuating Medicines, but they are always to be exhibited upon the maturest Consideration, and the best Advice. People that take up such Practices upon their own Opinions, will in the End find cause to repent it.

The best Way of curing the Gout, (if it may be allowed that Name) is to prevent it, that is, to hinder the Generation of this gouty Humour in the Body; this is to be effected no other way, that I know of, but by Diet: While the digestive Powers of the Body are in such full Strength and Vigour, as perfectly to assimilate the Food into its own Substance, and they be not oppressed with greater Loads than they are able to manage, the Choice of particular kinds of Diet will be of little Consequence; but these are always defective in gouty Persons, and these Defects are productive of different Habits in different Constitutions, which must be attended to in Rules for Diet in general, as well as in the Gout. Long Habits are not suddenly changeable with Safety; and after the *Ætas vergens*, the human Body doth not freely admit of Changes. A Body always supported in an high Manner, with Flesh Meats, and Wine, will not well bear a sudden Change to a low Diet; and on the contrary, a Body fed upon Water and Vegetables, will not well bear a sudden Change to an high Diet; sudden Repletions or Evacuation is dangerous, and therefore *Celsus* well advises, *Nullum cibi genus fugere, quo populus utatur, interdum in convictu esse, interdum ab eo se retrahere; modo plus justo, modo non amplius assumere*, but this is to be understood of People in Health.

Milk seems to be the best Medium of Diet, and yet from what was before said of it, there must be many gouty Constitutions it will not agree with; the same may be said of Turneps, which have been in their Day reckoned Specifick to the Gout as well as Milk; and the Truth is, that many Persons have suffered irreparable Damage, and some lost their Lives, by attempting particular Diets in improper Habits of Body. It is utterly disagreeable either to Reason or Experience, to fix any one general Rule of Diet that shall agree with all Constitutions, or even all gouty Constitutions. The particular Constitutions of gouty Persons are hardly reducible to general Rules, and nothing but Observations, and accurate Judgment, can determine upon them so as to direct a proper Diet. *Lewis Cornaro*, who is one of the strongest Instances of the force of Diet, in the little Account he hath published, tells us that he found several Particularities in his own Constitution, which his Physicians could no way satisfy him in. One Instance is much to our purpose, old Wine disagreed so much with him, that in the Months of *July* and *August*, in his later Years, he was forced to abstain altogether from Wine, this generally brought him to Death's Door every Year with perfect Weakness; for though he had been gouty, and cured of it by Diet, he never refrained from Flesh Meat or Wine in some small Quantities, nor could he relish or digest his Food without Wine: So soon as the Grapes began to turn, even before they were full Ripe, he had Wine pressed out for himself, whence he was wonderfully restored, in two or three Days, to the Admiration of his Physicians, who could not conceive, that new Wine, before thorough Defæcation, should have so good an Effect. *Cornaro* describes himself, and his own Diet very honestly;

but when he comes to give Rules for others, leaves the Kinds of Food to its Agreement or Disagreement to every particular Constitution; and concludes with this Maxim, which is undoubtedly true with Regard to Diet in general, That for such Persons, to whom no kind of Food is offensive, the Regulation of the Quantity, and not the Quality of the Food is principally to be attended to; in which this Rule is always to be strictly observed, that no greater Quantity even of the most proper Food, be taken at a Time, than the Stomach is very well able to digest.

Having premised thus much about the Regard to be had to particular Constitutions, in ascertaining a Diet in the Gout, we may very well enquire, what Diet is most proper to prevent the Collection of gouty Salts in the Juices of the Body? From what hath been already said, and from pretty certain Experience, we may conclude this to be the Milk of an healthy young Animal, fed upon Vegetables; the next eligible is a vegetable Diet; and if animal Diet be absolutely Necessary, (as no doubt, some Part of it may be to many Constitutions) the Flesh of such Animals, as feed upon Vegetables, is preferable to such as feed upon other Animals. I prefer Wines to vegetable Diet, because all fermented Liquors are produced from Vegetables; of these the softest and smoothest are always to be preferred to the harder and rougher, though none should be used farther than as an help to Digestion; for Water is the Drink proper to all Animals. To assign Reasons for these Assertions would be only to repeat what I have said before; for if that be true, these evidently follow from it.

But so it is, that through the Difference of Constitutions, or different Habits superinduced, many cannot bear a strict Attendance upon one kind of Food; it shall disagree with the Body, be nauseous to the Stomach, fail in giving proper Nourishment, or if too strictly persisted in, may Cure the Gout, and bring on some other more fatal Distemper, or bad Habit, and even this hath been the Case of Milk it self. It is not within the Compass of my present Design, nor indeed, I am afraid, within my Power to enumerate all the several different Constitutions of gouty Persons, and the different Modifications of Diet necessary for them: A Constitution that will bear living upon Bread and Milk, will no doubt be in an happier Way of being cured of the Gout, than one that cannot. But what will not bend, must not be broke; vegetable Food is too flatulent, and gives too little Nourishment to many Constitutions, who require Food already assimilated into animal Substance. Stomachs long used to Wine, require it in Digestion, and in many Cases and gouty Constitutions, even while a Cure is attempting by Diet, a little Flesh Meat must be allowed at certain Times, and the Powers of the Body kept up, by the Moderate use of Wine, chusing the easiest of Digestion, and the softest of each Kind; taking especial Care never to overload the digestive Powers, by too great Quantities; which is a Rule that will hold at all Times, and in all Constitutions; and is of so great Consequence, that if not attended to, it will invalidate the Force of any other Rules that can be given for Diet in the Gout, or any other Distemper.

The Necessity of varying from the strict Milk-Diet, in which the Cure of the Gout absolutely consists, according to the Unhappiness of particular gouty Constitutions; must be left to the Observations of the Patient, of the Agreement or Disagreement he shall have experienced of particular Kinds of Food, to his own Body; and to the Judgment and Advice of a skilful and diligent Physician.

CHAPTER. I.

Before I explain this Method of Cure, I would have my Reader take Notice, that he is not to expect any thing perfectly new: I only propose to confirm, by fresh Experience, what hath been long enough known. The Method of Cure here advanced consists in the proper Use of Milk for a Year and upwards. Many will perhaps wonder at my Endeavours to revive a Method so long known and exploded by Physicians, as hurtful to gouty Constitutions, and shortening the Period of Life itself: But being fully satisfied from Reason, and certain Experience, that this most excellent Remedy is the Gift of Providence, for the Relief of Persons afflicted with this cruel Distemper, I could not help drawing up and communicating my Experience and Observations for the Relief of others.

Cornelius Celsus, the celebrated *Roman* Physician, speaking of the Pains and Evil that gouty People suffer, tells us of some Persons who entirely avoided this Distemper by a strict Adherence to the Use of Asses Milk, and of others that by abstaining a whole Year from the Use of Wine and Women, were never afterwards troubled with it.

Among the Moderns, *John George Grezzell* hath wrote a very learned Treatise upon the Cure of the Gout by Milk, wherein many curious and useful Observations are delivered; that excellent Physician Dr. *James Sacks* hath inserted, in the *German* Ephemeris, a Method for the Use of Milk, communicated to him by a noble Baron, wherein many useful and elegant Observations, founded upon Experiment, are contained. The late learned *Waldsmid* hath published a learned Dissertation upon the Relief of gouty Persons by Milk, wherein he agrees with the Authors now mentioned as to the Cure. I have lately received a Letter from a *French* Gentleman my Friend, who having been for many Years afflicted in a most terrible Manner with the Gout, hath been now by the Use of Milk, free for some Years. From these Examples I had Occasion to admire the wonderful Effects of this Diet, and therefore advised it to many gouty Persons here at *Cassell*, who have all recovered a perfect State of Health, by a strict Adherence to the Regimen Necessary in the Use of this Remedy: Even some whose Limbs were before perfectly crippled, are now able to walk and exercise. Colonel *Nicholas Dumont* hath experienced the Efficacy of this Method here at *Cassell*, for his Limbs were so entirely contracted that he was forced to use Crutches, but having confined himself strictly to the Use of this Diet for an Year and an half, he walks very well without a Cane, and hath performed several Journies. I have been free from the Gout my self upwards of an Year, notwithstanding I had three or four Fits every Year for Sixteen foregoing. Colonel *Haste* hath been restored by the same Means, though he hath had some mild Returns at several Times.

I shall in the first Place communicate the Letter I just now mentioned; next I shall lay down the Rules Necessary to be observed in the Use of this Milk-Diet; I shall then demonstrate from undeniable Principles, that this Method is the most convenient to asswage and cure the Gout, and that no bad Consequences can attend the Constitution, if it be taken with the proper Regulations. The Letter is as Follows.

To Monsieur de Collet.

SIR,

Nothing can be more agreeable to me, than to satisfy the Desire of my Friends afflicted with the Gout, in communicating the Method of Diet, by which the Marquis *de Bongi, Mons. Chamar,* and my self were relieved from the Gout; you will please to take Notice, that the Milk we used was fresh drawn from the Cow, Morning and Evening, without other Art than that we both eat and supped it, as warm as we could well bear it; my Reason for mentioning eating and supping the Milk, is, because as soon as we arose in the Morning we supped a large Bowl of warm Milk; but the Milk which was brought us at Dinner and Supper, we eat with fine light Bread, cut thin and put therein; this is all our Secret in this Matter. Persons afflicted with the Gout may promise themselves Relief, provided that once a Month, during the Course of this Diet, or at least once in two Months, they take a gentle Purge, which we made Use of, and were so strict in our Regimen, that we neither drank Wine nor, eat other Food, than Biscuits made of very fine Flower, Eggs, and Sugar, and some sweet Fruits, as Strawberries in Summer, but we chiefly avoided Raspberries. For my own Part, I never sweetned my Milk with Sugar, though some Friends who were in the same Course did, yet without any bad Effect. The Marquis *de Bongi* used to mix Crabs Eyes with his Milk before Dinner, upon a Presumption, that it would prevent any Sourness in his Stomach, but neither Monsieur *Chamar* or I ever used that Remedy. When we had strictly adhered to this Diet for a Year, we began to hope we might eat Fish, or indulge our Appetites in some varieties of Food, which one or other of us did, more or less, occasionally, and without any bad Effects. At the End of Nine Months I apprehended my Stomach to be somewhat weakened, which made me resolve to use a Glass of Wine after my Milk, and accordingly after Dinner and Supper every Day, I drank one Glass of Wine, in which I sopped a bit of Bread; this was very delicious to me while I used it. At length as we found the State of our Healths to mend, we began to eat and drink with our Friends. This Method hath succeeded so well, that we live hitherto in our common Way upon Milk, yet not so strictly, but that we dine or sup, once, twice or thrice a Week with our Friends in their Manner, and return afterwards to our Milk without Ceremony; and by the Blessing of God we are wonderfully well. We dont here pretend to say, that none of us have been since afflicted with the Gout, for the Marquiss *de Bongi* hath had two or three pretty sharp Fits; but both he and I know the Difference between having two or three Fits in nine or ten Years, and of being perpetually oppressed, and confined to Bed with this cruel Distemper, which was our Case before; especially the Marquiss *de Bongi*, who at Six and Thirty was almost continually confined to his Bed, deprived of the Use of his Limbs, and the Joints of his Hands and Feet knotted and chalky; instead of which, he now uses his Limbs without any Marks of Infirmity, insomuch that any one who had seen him in his former bad State, and compares it with his present, would look on him as one raised from Death to Life. As for Monsieur *Chamar*, and my self, who are more advanced in Years, considering our Age, we are mighty well; 'tis true indeed that sometimes, as upon Changes of Weather, or of the Moon, we find (or at least we fancy so) that we have some Threatnings of Pain, especially about those Joints where the Gout used to ravage, but a little Exercise soon dissipates those Apprehensions.

It is now Seven Years, that Monsieur *Chamar* and I have adhered to this Diet, in all which Time we have neither of us been so far oppressed by the Gout, as to be confined to our Beds, or even to our Chambers, so much as one whole Day; notwithstanding before we fell into this Method (though we were not perpetually under actual Fits of the Gout) we had a continued Weakness in our Limbs, we walked very infirmly and with difficulty, and if we chanced to make a wrong Step, or to slip in walking, we suffered Extremity of Pain; our Case is now so far altered, that we walk as firm, as if we had never had the Gout. I must confess indeed that both the Marquiss and I used the Diet for a good while, before we perceived any manifest Change, but afterwards our Pain diminished by Degrees, and the Strength of our Limbs returned. The Milk must be used a good while, that the natural Temper and Vigour of the Constitution may have Time and Leisure to come to itself; for though this Diet may be often used Six Months or even Twelve before the Patient can use his Limbs free from Pain, yet let him not despair, for if once he begins to gather Strength, it will daily increase. As to Purging, and Evacuation of the Humours, if possible it should be done once a Month, in the Decrease of the Moon: I hold purging extremely Necessary; for my own Part, it was what I did for the first Seven or Eight Months of this Diet constantly, till I grew tired of it. This is truly the Method I used, and though I afterwards remitted, I found no bad Consequence. The Marquiss and I, at present, take a Bowl of Warm

Milk every Morning, but for the Rest of the Day drink and eat as usual. The Marquiss indeed, for the Space of Eight Years, hath had at Times several small Fits of the Gout, but for my self I have hardly had any, except sometimes upon Changes of the Weather, or of the Moon, I have perceived a Numbness and Weakness in my Knees and Joints, like Threatenings of the Gout; but I thank God, it never confined me, and as it came on easily, it as easily went off. The following is the Method of purging: *Take of Scammony, white Turbith, Hermodactyls, Leaves of Sena, Sarsaparilla, Cinamon, and Sugar, of each one Drachm, powder them very fine, and divide the whole into Seven equal Parts, one of which is a Dose, and may be taken in white wine or a little Broth.* It is necessary to purge once a Month, especially in the Decline of the Moon. If it be thought necessary to purge twice in the Month, let the first Dose be taken in the last Quarter, the second the last Day of the Quarter. The Day I took Physick, I used Milk after it as usual. When I had pursued this Course about Seven or Eight Months, I found my Stomach so much weakened from the Milk, that I was forced to take a Glass of Red Wine every Day after Dinner, which agreed mighty well with me, and I have continued it ever since; so that I am often impatient to finish my Milk, that I may have the Pleasure of regaling my self with a Glass of Wine, and a bit of Bread.

CHAPTER. II.

In the foregoing Letter are contained many useful Observations about the Use of Milk, and its wonderful Efficacy in the Cure of the Gout, from uncontestable Facts, in the Account of the Persons there named. I shall next lay down the Method of this Diet, by which many Persons here at *Cassell* were relieved. Whoever expects Benefit by this Method, must observe the following Rules. No one ought to go into this Diet without having his Body duly prepared; he must take Care by Degrees to change his Habit, and for the first Month to regulate his Diet, by strictly avoiding all Salt or smoaked Meats; Legumes, and stale, acid or feculent Liquors, and to eat white Meats sparingly, with clear small Drink, as small Beer or Barley Water, or Decoctions of the Woods: A Glass of *Moselle* or *French* Wine free from Acidity, may be allowed at Dinner, and Gruels and Broths made of white Meats. There is a necessary Caution to be used, that both in Meat and Drink, the Quantity taken be rather within the Appetite than beyond it; for from overloading the digestive Powers, arise Crudities, Flatulencies, and acid Humours, which are the Origine of many Disorders. Upon this Account it is necessary to purge the Bowels, two or three Times a Month, with Tincture of Jalap, Elixir *Proprietatis*, Rhubarb, some of the purging Pills, as the Arthritick or Mastich Pills; that the Viscidity arising from indigestions may be carried forth of the Bowels, and the Stomach be better disposed to receive and digest the Milk. I am of Opinion, the first Dose should be taken the first Day of the Month, preparatory to this Diet, the second after some few Weeks of this first Regimen, and the third the last Day of the Month; after this I advice the taking an Ounce of Crabs-Eyes, or prepared calcined Hartshorn, especially if there yet remains any Marks of Acidity in the first Passages. This further Caution is very absolutely Necessary, that not only in the first Month, but in all subsequent, all Passion, chiefly Anger and Grief be avoided, because of their pernicious Consequences; more especially the Use of Women during the whole Year.

SECT. 2.

All those who have other Distempers complicated with the Gout, as the Scurvy, Leprosy, bad Habit of Body, Stone or Gravel, Hystericks, the Pox, or other Distemper arising from the Impurity of the Blood, too great a viscidity or acrimony of the Juices, or a known or latent Acid in the Blood, are first to use Absorbent, Diuretick, Sweetening or other Medicines, proper to their particular Distempers, till the Acrimony or Tenacity of the Blood and Humours be corrected, the Acid expelled, and such complicated Disorders overcome, and then apply this noble Remedy of a Milk-Diet to the Cure of the Gout alone, from which they may certainly promise themselves Success: But if while the Body is ill prepared, or full of vitiated Juices, the Milk-Diet should be preposterously brought into Use, they will not only be disappointed in their hopes of Relief, but bring certain Destruction, and Increase of their Disorders; as actually happened to the Count *de Perlebourgh*, and *a Lubech* Consul in this Neighbourhood, who having a Complication of Distempers, made an improper Trial of a Milk-Diet.

SECT. 3.

The Milk in which the Cure of the Gout consists, ought to be excellent in its Kind; the Animal from whence it is taken, as described by *Waldsmid*, should be an Heifer, or Cow of a middle Age, of a good Habit, either of Red or a Black Colour, (though this need not so strictly be minded) neither fat nor lean, nor pregnant, and kept separate from the Bull: In Winter fed upon good Hay, Barley, Bran or Straw; in Summer at good Grass, and led in a Collar like an Horse. If any one can keep a Cow for their own Use, it is best, and they may more safely rely upon help from it; but if not, the Milk as the Milkmen sell it will do; taking Care however that the Cow be of a good Habit, well fed, and not too old.

SECT. 4.

As to the Quality and Quantity of the Milk, it is to be observed, that as soon as it is milked it should be warmed, but not so as to boil it. Let the Vessel full of Milk be put into boiling Water, and when it is so hot as to be conveniently supped, or at least so warm as when it came from the Cow, let it be taken after the Manner of Tea or Coffee. The Times of taking ought to be, two Pints in the Morning, some four or Five Hours before Dinner, as much about Noon, and as much about Seven in the Evening; but the Quantity cannot be exactly determined, because the Weakness or Strength of the Stomach must give a Rule in this Case; or let so much be taken as the Stomach can bear without Inconvenience, and the Patient may increase the Quantity daily till he comes to about forty Ounces. If the Stomach be weak, he may take it in a smaller Quantity, four or five Times a Day; if four Times, let two of them serve for Dinner and Supper, with some of the finest wheaten Bread; and a Draught of Milk may be repeated every four Hours; if the Milk be taken at five Times, it may be so ordered as to let three Hours intervene; those who are of more robust Constitutions, may be content with three Meals of Milk a Day; and it will not be amiss to take every Morning a Dose of Crabs-Eyes, or some other absorbent Powder: I usually take about twelve or fourteen Ounces of Milk in the Morning, Twenty four Ounces with Wheat Bread at Noon, and about Twenty Ounces at Night, half with Bread, and the other half drank as common

Drink. Some allow the Use of white Meats at Dinner, lessening the Quantities by Degrees, and making up the Deficiencies by Food of Milk and Eggs, so that by Degrees the Milk and Eggs are entirely substituted in the Place of the Flesh Meat, and then by diminishing the Eggs daily, Milk becomes entirely substituted for other Food: This Method seems to me, entirely agreeable to tender Constitutions, and such as dont well bear sudden Changes. Some who have strictly adhered to Milk for fourteen Weeks, have indulged in the Use of poached Eggs without Salt, Barley boiled in Milk, fresh Butter without Salt, Custard and other Milk Foods; and in Summer, some Kinds of Fruits, as Strawberries, Peaches, &c. tho' in my Judgment improperly, especially such Fruits as are cold, or seem to have a latent Acid, or such as weaken the Bowels. On this Head it may be observed in general, that the less whatever be used for Food differs in its Nature from Milk, it may be more freely ventured upon in the Milk-Diet; but the Prudence and Care of the Physician is to be relied on, according to the Diversity of Circumstances that may happen in different Constitutions.

SECT. 5.

This Diet ought to be so long continued, until the whole gouty Matter be discharged forth of the Body, which is to be computed by the Degree and Length of the Distemper, and Observations upon the Cure in others. The longer it is continued, the more perfect Cure is to be expected; those that are over-run with the Distemper, are always to use it, others for an Year, and others for an Year and an half; some Persons who have, upon continuing it only for half an Year, thought themselves perfectly cured, and have returned too soon to their former Method of living, have so far exceeded, as to be seized again with the Gout, but returning to the Diet, have been cured; some more prudent, have continued the Diet for an Year, and then returned to their ordinary Manner of living by Degrees, always taking about sixteen Ounces or a Pint of Milk every Morning, and have thus for many Years been free. The best Time of Beginning the Diet is in the Spring, and that from the Beginning of *May*, to the End of *April* in the succeeding Year.

SECT. 6.

Some have in the Continuance of this Diet been seized with Oppressions and Difficulty of Breathing, Weakness in their Limbs, Coughs and Phlegm; but these Symptoms either vanish of themselves, or quickly give way to Elixir *Proprietatis* without an Acid, Spirit of Hartshorn succinated, *Sal volatile oleosum*, or any of the more fixed absorbent alkaline Medicines.

SECT. 7.

For those who are oppressed with an abundance of Humours, whose Bowels are full of Flatulencies, or are constipated, let them once in every Month or Six Weeks take a gentle Purge of Rhubarb, or of the Arthritick Pills, or half a Scruple of *Pill Ruffi*, or of *Sylvius* his Gum Pills: But if the Body be open, and the Milk passes too quickly through, it may suffice to take twenty Grains of Rhubarb; or if the Body be bound, take twenty Grains of Rhubarb in the first Draught of Milk, drinking the rest of the Quantity after it, or else in the Evening take twenty Drops of the Essence of Rhubarb with the Milk, and repeat it as often as there may be Occasion; but for the general, if it can be conveniently done, the purging Medicines should be used in the Decrease of the Moon.

SECT. 8.

If the Milk should occasion a Looseness, let it boil before it is used, adding a Grain of Salt and so supping it hot; if it do not succeed the first Time, try it a second Time, and a third; but if it doth not do then, take a Dose of Crabs-Eyes, *Unicornu fossile*, or *Terra sigillata*.

SECT. 9.

If the Milk should heat the Body, let a third Part of Barley Water, made with Raisins, be added to it; or if it occasion Thirst at any Time, Barley Water with Raisins; or in case of a Cough, the pectoral Decoction may be used between the Intervals of using the Milk.

SECT. 10.

If the Stomach be weakened by the Use of the Milk, the Patient may be allowed Sugar Biscuits, sopped in *Spanish*, *Italian* or *Burgundy* Wine, or any other that is neither Acid nor Foul; and if necessary, even a Glass of those Wines: Thus the Stomach will be fortified, and more easily perform its Office; if there should be a Necessity for it, some of the warm aromatic Powders may be brought into Use.

SECT. 11.

After this Diet hath been used twelve or fourteen Months, the Patient may begin to use Flesh Meats of easy Digestion, avoiding sharp, acid or salt Meats, but using such as we mentioned before, drinking Milk still, or small Beer well wrought, neither stale nor turbid.

SECT. 12.

The Cure being thus absolutely finished, it will be still necessary to take every Morning a Pint of warm Milk, and to be constantly cautious about your Diet, avoiding every thing acid or sharp.

SECT. 13.

To prevent the Milk from cruddling, some Sugar may be mixed with it, or even a little Salt, thus the Acid is prevented from gathering; but this should be done but seldom, and upon the most urgent Necessity.

SECT. 14.

Though there should not follow an immediate or sensible Change upon the Use of the Milk for some Time, yet the Patient ought not to be disheartned; for if these Rules be strictly observed, and the Patient be otherwise in a good Habit, the Pains will vanish by Degrees, and a due Strength and Tone return to the Limbs.

CHAPTER. III.

I Have now delivered the Directions I proposed, partly from the
Authors before-mentioned, and partly from my own Experience; by a due
Observation of which many Persons have been perfectly relieved from this
grievous Distemper; of which I shall give some Examples. *D. Sorbait*, p.
741, tells us, that he knew several Persons, by the Use of the Milk-Diet,
either perfectly cured, or their Gout so much overcome, that their Pains
were dwindled to nothing. *John Pilus*, the Emperour's Surgeon told me, that
tho' he frequently had Fits of the Gout, and almost lost the Use of his
Limbs, so that he was in a very miserable Condition, yet for these three
Years past, by the Help of this Diet, he hath been perfectly free from Pain,
his Countenance is now become fresh and healthy, he hath had several
Children, and appears as if he were born a-new. Count *Coningseck*, his
Imperial Majesty's Counsellour, found the same Benefit by this Diet; and
Count *S. Hillario* of the Emperour's Bed-Chamber; several others, who
were almost worn out with the Gout, grown pale and wan, have in a
manner become young and florid again by this Diet. The Bishop of
Wallendorf, tho' quite impotent by the Gout, was cured by Milk. Three noble
French Refugees, the Marquess *de Bongi*, Monsieur *de Chamar*, and the
Counsellour *de Talo*, have been now many Years free from the Gout, as
appears by the Letter before inserted. I am told that a Consul, and several
others at *Hambourgh*, are now using this Diet with Success. A Counsellour
of *Oldenbourgh*, the Sieur *Van Velden*, hath used this Diet this last Winter
with very wonderful Success; for tho' he could neither use his Hands nor
Feet, he uses both now readily and perfectly well. A Miner here in the
Neighbourhood hath used Milk for these six Months past with great
Benefit; he was almost a cripple, but now walks very well to the Mines. All
the World knows that the famous Prince of *Conde* was cured of the Gout in
France by Milk-Diet. There are two Citizens of *Hambourgh*, one of which,
tho' he hath had the Gout fifteen Years, is well recovered by the Use of
Milk, and the Knots in his Joints are quite wore away. Colonel *Haste* hath
used Milk for six Months, and been free from the Gout; and tho' he hath
left off the Use of it, the Fits are much easier than before. There is no
Occasion to multiply Examples; many more may be found in *Sorbait, Sacks,
Greizel, Waldsmid*, Authors already named. I have experienced the great
Benefit of this Diet in myself; I was so cruelly handled by this Distemper,
that I almost lost the Use of my Limbs, and at last had a Fit every Month or
Six Weeks; I was at the same Time violently afflicted with the Stone, and
difficulty of Urine; but now that I have confined myself to this Diet for an
Year and upwards, I have not only been free from any Fit in that Time, but

the Strength of my Limbs is returned, the Dysury is abated; and what is wonderful, the Stone in my Bladder is lessened and dissolving, so that I now hope I shall get the better of the Gout, having been in a manner free from it an Year and an half; I have had some Fits indeed, but very mild ones. I take Milk to be a Medicine beyond any yet discovered for the Stone, since within the Space of one Year, the Stone in my Bladder diminished an Ounce, as I judge from the Bits I have voided and collected in that Time; and since I have left off the Cure, I have not voided one Bit. I am of Opinion, contrary to most Physicians, that Milk doth not breed the Stone in the Bladder, but only a viscid kind of Phlegm in that or any other Part.

SECT. 2.

These Things premised, I shall next examine how it comes to pass that Milk is endued with this mighty Power; but it is necessary first to enquire concerning the genuine Cause of the Gout. All the Symptoms testify the first and nearest Cause to be some viscid, sharp Liquor, endued with some acid or lixivial corrosive Salt, more or less fixed; this Salt indeed occasions such a singular smart Pain, that it seems to be specifick. I think it not only acid, but also somewhat austere, from the different earthy, cheesy Particles it contains. Hence it fixes its sharp stiff Points in the Membranes, Tendons and Nerves, and more readily thickens and coagulates the lymphatick Juices. Where and how this Liquor that causes the Gout is generated, I shall explain in a few Words. First then the Stomach and Bowels, whether from too great an use of Wine or Women, or from too sedentary a Life, and want of due Exercise, or from the particular Disposition of the stomachick Juices, or from bad Diet, become so affected, that by Degrees the Digestion or Dissolution of the Food is lessened; the Chyle thence produced, becomes more thick and viscid than formerly; so that this Chyle, thus delivered into the Blood, renders its Mass thicker, and of Consequence the several Secretions of the Humours, as the Lymph, animal Spirits, the mucilaginous Juices about the Joints are more slowly performed; thus the Stomach and Bowels become more tainted, the stomachick Juices and those separated by the Glands of the Intestines become more viscid, and the Difficulty of Digestion is increased; Part of the Food turns to Flatulency, and viscid sharp Slime in the Bowels; Part of the Chyle becomes infected with a corrosive acid Salt thence produced, and being again thrown into the Blood, the Lymph and other Juices become infected with the same acid Salt, which gives Birth to many Distempers. It is observable these viscid Juices, thus stopped in their Progress, and infected with this noxious Salt, so as to be more liable to an intestine than a progressive Motion, are the most subject to Corruption of any in the Body, and to contract a Thickness, and Inaptitude to Motion. Such an Humour is the Lymph, and more especially the mucilaginous Juice separated in the Glands of the

Joints, in order to keep them moist and smooth for Motion. If therefore a sufficient Quantity of these acid Salts be brought into the Mass of the Blood, or the Humours impregnated with them, be lodged about the nervous or tendinous Membranes, and there acquire so extraordinary a Tenacity or Sharpness, as to be coagulated, the Gout thence arises, as is evident both from Reason and Experience. That this may more evidently appear, I shall next explain the Figure, Situation and Structure of these Glands.

SECT. 3.

These Glands, as described by Dr. *Havers* in his new Osteology, and as they discover themselves upon Dissection, are of two Kinds; some are small and thickly interspersed in the Membranes of the Joints, and with very few Exceptions of an equal Bigness, so as to render the Membrane perfectly Glandulous: In some Parts of the Membrane, in the Joints, and in the Furrows of the Bone, these Glands are so united as to form very remarkable and large conglomerate Glands. In some of the large Joints there is but one, as in the Hip Joint; in others, as in the Knee, four or five; they are of a red Colour, which is communicated from the blood Vessels; as to their Substance, soft and papillary, tho' not tender and friable; they are in their Structure Conglomerate, consisting of divers Membranes, wove one within another, interspersed with small round Vesicles, which are not only contiguous, but adhere closely one to another, as the Membranes also do. By the Pores of these little Vesicles a mucilaginous Liquor is strained and secerned from the general Mass of the arterial Blood, and thence by the excretory Duct, with which all these Glands are furnished, is shed into the Interstices of all the Joints.

SECT. 4.

These Glands have a sufficient Number of blood Vessels, they dont come out of them in right Lines, but are observed to have many Convolutions, Windings, and Insertions; there seems to be a very particular Reason, from the Nature of the Liquor to be separated, for this Obliquity of the blood Vessels; for since that Liquor is to be viscid and mucilaginous, its Parts should proceed slowly, and not without Difficulty, through the glandulary Pores; and therefore the Vessels are contorted in the Manner we see, that the Motion of the Blood may be retarded, and more Time and Leizure given, both for the separating Particles of such a Nature, and for their Admission through the Pores of the Glands.

SECT. 5.

These Glands are of different Shapes, so as to fit the Furrows and Cavities where they are placed; some are long, others conical, broad at their

Base and grow narrow towards the Top, so as to terminate in an Edge; some have a broad Base, and rise into a sort of Cone; some are like little Ridges; some like Fringe; some are broad and pretty flat.

SECT. 6.

As to their Situation, they are differently seated in the several Joints; in some they stand over-against the very Interstice of the Bones, and run in a little way between them, where the Ends of the Bones towards that Side are not contiguous, but so formed as in their Conjunction to make an Interstice, and these are commonly in the Manner of a Fringe; some are seated in some Sinus or Cavity, others planted upon the Membrane, which immediately covers the Articulation: In general they are so seated, that they cannot be injured by a Compression from the Bones; and yet there is this Contrivance, that the Bone does, either in the Inflexion or Extension of the Joint, lightly press upon them, so as to promote the Excretion of the Humour, which they separate into the Joints, when they are moved and stand most in need of it; and by this Means it seems to be most plentifully supplied, when there is occasion for the greatest Quantity of it, and to be proportioned to the present Exigence, according to the State of Rest, or the several Degrees of Motion in the Part when it is moved. And it is no small Security to these Glands, against the Obstructions which the mucilaginous Quality of the Liquor that they separate does naturally dispose them to, that they are solicited, and the Liquor expressed out of them by the Motion of the Parts where they are seated: The same sort of Glands are placed about the common Membrane of the Muscles, and about the Tendons.

SECT. 7.

The Liquor that is separated from these Glands is a Mucilage, not unlike the White of an Egg, tho' not always so clear and pellucid; when pure it is very like it. In some Animals it is of a Colour inclining to Yellow, and is composed of watry, saline and slimy Particles; it is supposed that the earthy Particles may be about a two and thirtieth Part. The Nature of this Mucilage seems nearly to approach to that of the *Serum* of the Blood, separated from the grumous Part upon being exposed to the Air, and exhibit much the same Appearances upon Trials by Mixture with other Bodies, only the *Serum* is not so mucilaginous. The *Serum* is coagulated upon being mixed with Spirit or Oyl of Vitriol, Spirit of Salt, Oyl of Sulphur, and other acid Spirits. The *Serum*, upon being held in a Spoon over the Fire, becomes a thick Jelly, and at length a sort of friable Glew; on the contrary, the Mucilage grows thinner, upon the same Application, throws up a slight thin Film at Top, and produces but a slight Coagulum. After the aqueous Parts are evaporated, there remains scarce a thirtieth Part of the whole Mass.

SECT. 8.

The principal Use of this Mucilage is to lubricate the Joints, and to render and preserve the Extremities of the Bones, at their Articulations, smooth and supple, for the easy Performance of animal Motion. Besides this mucilaginous Liquor from these Glands, there is an oily medullary kind of Substance transmitted through the very Bone into the Cavity of the Joints: These two Liquors are mixed by the Motion of the Joints, the Mucilage contributes to make the Oyl more slimy, and the Oyl preserves the Mucilage from stiffening into a Jelly. This Mucilage further serves to prevent the Extremities of the Joints from being burnt up in the Gout. In the same Manner the Muscles and Tendons are lubricated and kept in Vigour by the Liquor supplied from the same kind of Glands placed on their Membranes.

SECT. 9.

This Mucilage is formed from the purer Part of the Lymph and the serous Parts of the Blood, and separated in these Glands from the Mass of the Blood. In order to have a more distinct Notion of its constituent Parts, and to know how it comes to occasion the Gout, the following Experiments of Dr. *Havers* may be very properly repeated in this Place. He made most of the Trials both when it was hot and when it was cold. Vinegar dropt into it, when it was hot, made a considerable Coagulation with a *Serum*; it must be observed that those Mixtures that were made with it cold, did produce the same Effect when it was warmed, namely a Coagulation with Acids and Stypticks, only in an higher Degree: And whereas the Coagulations, which were made when it was in one State, did only change it into a thick Jelly without any *Serum*, after the Manner of a Cheese when it is newly set, as they term it, which over the Fire afterwards exhibited two distinct Parts, a *Coagulum* and a Whey; in the other, that is, when the Mucilage was hot, the Mixtures which coagulated it produced an harder Curd, and a *Serum* distinct from it. By dropping in some of the Decoction of Galls into it, the whole turned into a gelatinous Mass, and it was all a Sort of *Coagulum* like a Skin, of a whitish Colour, and so tough as to hang all together when it was taken up with a Needle. This *Coagulum* or Jelly being laid in the Sun, and dried, the Parts of it stuck all together in one Piece, but was very friable and easily rubbed to a Powder, which was very much like fine Flower. The same Effect had the strong Infusion of Balaustia, red Roses, Pomegranate Bark, and the *Peruvian* Bark, although there was some Difference in the Coagulation, according to the different Degrees of their Astringency. With a few Drops of *Aqua Fortis* distilled upon it, the Mucilage was immediately coagulated, though the *Coagulum*, which was white, was so tender, that it would by Agitation be dissolved in fair Water, and make it of the same Colour almost like Milk; Spirit of Nitre made exactly the same Alteration in it as *Aqua Fortis* did, a *Coagulum* which was of a white Colour. Vinegar, Spirit of Salt of Vitriol, Oyl of Vitriol, and of Sulphur in some Mucilage which I tried it with, did not make any considerable Alteration when it was cold, but in some other it did more; when *Aqua Fortis* and Spirit of Nitre did produce in all the same Effects in the same Degree. It was mighty observable, that so strong an Acid as Oyl of Vitriol should have no greater Effect upon it to alter it not, so considerable as that of Vinegar, which would incline one to think that it is not always the high Degree of Acidity that works this Change. But there seems to be something particular in Wines, which disposes them to coagulate this Liquor, when any of them are made Use of; and those Parts of them, which are apt to act thus upon it, are cast into those Interstices where they have the Mucilage singly to work upon. And therefore we find how readily any Wines do procure the Paroxysms of the Gout, where the Tone of the Glands is weakned, and the Patient hath a Disposition to this Distemper; which agrees with those Trials I have made with some of them: For Claret, white Wine, and even Sack, but the Claret especially, did make a *Coagulum* like a Jelly; and it was not strange that Claret, which hath both an Acid and a Stypticity in it, should produce the greatest Coagulation. A mercurial Water made of Sublimate and *Aqua Calcis*, made a very considerable whitish Coagulation, and rendred it all a thick Jelly, which being held over the Fire, turned to a Curd and a *Serum*. A Solution of *Roman* Vitriol produced a Coagulation likewise; so did Allum dissolved in Water, but it made a greater Alteration in some than it did in others, though the Mucilages were taken from subjects of the same Species. *Saccharum Saturni* did inspissate it, which appeared to be a true Coagulation, because with the Fire they would turn to a distinct *Coagulum* and *Serum*. Salt of Wormwood made no sensible Alteration, only it seemed a little thicker, to which I put some of the Decoction of Galls, which immediately produced a Coagulation. Upon dropping in some Spirit of Vitriol, to see what would be the Effect of the Colluctation of the Salt and Spirit, and I found, after it was over, that the *Coagulum* and the serous Part were distinguished, and the *Serum* limpid like Water. I took some of the Decoction of Galls, and added to it Spirit of Vitriol, intending to make a strong Acid austere, where I observed that these two by themselves produced a strong Coagulation; and stirring of them together, to see if the whole might not be brought to mix by that Means, I found the *Coagulum* turned into a viscous Body, and a perfect soft Gum. Then I took out the Gum, and poured some Mucilage to the residuous Liquor, by which it was changed so as to assume a whitish Colour, but was not considerably coagulated; which it was the less, because the austere Parts were most of them, with some of the Acid, precipitated into the Gum which had been separated from the serous Part. But if the Spirit of Vitriol and the Mucilage are first mixed, and the austere Liquor be afterwards added, they make a very considerable and plentiful *Coagulum*, which will only be broken into smaller Parts, and not be dissolved in Water. *Aqua Fortis*, and the Decoction of Galls being both dropt into some of the Mucilage, made a white *Coagulum*, which likewise was not dissolved in Water, altho' with *oleum Tartari per Deliquium*, and so with Spirit of *Sal Ammoniac* dropt into it, I presently dissolved it. I found likewise, that the *Coagulum* made with the Infusion of Pomegranate Peel, red Roses and Balaustia, being mixed with some of the Mucilage, to which an Acid had been put, made the *Coagulum* more firm, so that it would not dissolve in fair Water; but yet the Oyl of Tartar by *Deliquium*, and the Spirit of *Sal Ammoniac*, did the Business in all of them. The *Coagulum* of the Mucilage made with an Acid, and the Infusion of the *Peruvian* Bark and several other Astringents, I kept and dried, which when they were first put to the Teeth, seemed a little gritty, though after they were moist they were of a softer Nature. All the Mixtures made of the Mucilage with an Acid and an Austere, produced not only a plentiful Coagulation of a white Colour, but such a one as was of a thicker Consistence, and not Soluble in fair Water, as that was which was made with an Acid only.

CHAPTER. IV.

It is now proper to apply what hath been hitherto delivered, to the Distemper we are treating of, that from thence the Powers of Milk in the Cure may more clearly appear. We have shewed before how the Mass of the Blood becomes impregnated with a saline Acrimony, more or less Acid, from a sharp and indigested Chyle, and the Powers of Digestion weakned and impaired; whence is easily explained how the Lymph and acrid *Serum* is communicated to the mucilaginous Glands, and the smallest Branches of the Arteries, so as to infect and coagulate the Mucilage, in Proportion to the Quantity of Salts they contain. The Fibres of the Membranes and Tendons are vellicated by the Acrimony of those Salts, so as to occasion intolerable Pain, and affect the Nerves to a very great Degree.

SECT. 2.

From the Diversity of Pains and other Symptoms in the Gout, it appears that these saline Particles are sometimes salt and pungent, sometimes more volatile, sharp and burning. That the mucilaginous Humour is frequently acid and corrosive in the Gout, appears from hence, that this Liquor is neither so easily coagulated, nor acquires so great a Degree of Viscidity by any other Mixture as with austere Acids, and from the Obstinacy and Duration of the Pain. It is frequently observed, that upon the Approach of a Fit, People complain of sowre Belchings, Wind, and vomit acid Humours, so that hypochondriac People, and such as are subject to the Gravel, are most apt to be seized with this Distemper; this may afford a good Reason why not only the drinking of acid Wines bring on a Fit in gouty Persons, but originally occasion the Gout in such Persons as frequently drink them. The Mixture of Wine with the Mucilage plainly evinces, that the acid Particles of the Wine give a Disposition to the Distemper, for it caused a greater Coagulation of the Mucilage than Oyl of Vitriol, whence easily appears what Mischief it may do to gouty Persons.

SECT. 3.

How this sharp acid Humour comes to be secerned in the Glands, seems to want Explanation, and this I judge to be in the following Manner. The Blood being first imbued with a sufficient Quantity of these saline heterogeneous Particles, which it receives from the corrupted Chyle, is by Degrees disturbed in its Motion, and the Fibres of the Nerves begin to be sensibly irritated, so as to cause irregular Motions of the animal Spirits. The Blood itself is thickned, because these saline and viscid Particles get into the small Ramifications of the Arteries, and occasion Obstructions there; by this Means the natural Functions and Secretions of the Humours, especially in the Glands, are disturbed, and proceed slower; and accordingly for some Time before the Fit, we find Complaints of Crudities in the Stomach, a swelling and Heaviness of Body, and Weakness and Numbness of the Limbs, which increase daily till the Fit is formed. At length the Blood, by continued Irritations, being put into more violent Motions, drives these saline heterogeneous viscid Particles through the obstructed Capillaries into the glandular Vesicles, whence without doubt the Juices there secerned, especially that of which we are speaking, *viz.* the Mucilage in the Glands in and about the Joints, is not only plentifully stored with these acid corrosive Salts, becomes more viscid and ropy, but also very corrosive and poignant; and while it irritates and corrodes the adjoining Membranes and Tendons, not only causes violent Pains, but also since by the Contraction of the Nerves the Blood cannot move so freely through the smallest Vessels, the Fibres are distended, and an inflammatory Tumor frequently succeeds.

SECT. 4.

The Reason why the Gout affects particularly the Hands and Feet, and not all the Joints together, where Glands of the same Nature are placed, seems to be this: The Blood vitiated in the Manner before explained, propelling these saline Parts into the Pores of the Glands, from the inequality of its Motion in the Time of a Fit, does not impel those Salts with an equable Force, but chiefly into such Parts (especially the Feet and other pendulous Members) where the Pressure and Impulse lies heaviest; so dilates the Cavities of the smallest Canals, till at length it deposits Part of such Salts, with other viscid Humours, upon those Glands. Thus being partly freed from those Salts, the Gout does not seize other Parts with the same Violence; for frequently a large Quantity of such vitiated Humours are secerned by Urine, Sweat, and other more open Passages; and it even often happens, that Persons whose Juices are much corrupted, have avoided the Distemper by the Laxity and Openness of their Vessels; yet these very Persons, when the Blood becomes oppressed by these saline Particles in so great Degree, as not to be readily discharged by the larger Passages, they affect the Mucilage in the Glands and occasion the Gout.

SECT. 5.

That this Distemper comes by Fits, appears owing to this, that upon the Approach of a Fit much of the morbifick Matter is thrown upon the Glands by the Blood, so that the Blood thus freed from sharp and viscid Particles, moves easier and freer, till such Time as a sufficient Quantity of morbifick Matter is again generated in the Blood; which by separating again, a viscid and sharp Mucilage, the Symptoms of the Gout, are repeated in another Fit. The feverish Chilliness and Shivering that attends the Gout, is to be accounted for from the irregular Motion of the Blood, occasioned by the Salt and viscid Particles; and it is very likely that those very Salts themselves, irritating the Nerves, and occasioning inordinate and violent Motions of the animal Spirits, contribute to such a Fever; this Sharpness of the Blood, while the Salts are thrown forth by Urine or Sweat, remits till the Blood be again infected. We observe that the Gout often prevents other Distempers; for by this Expulsion of the corrupted Parts from the Blood, Distempers which might have arisen from them are prevented.

SECT. 6.

Because there is a great Difference made between the fixed and wandering Gout, I shall observe a few Things thereon. As to the wandering Gout, it is observable that the Mucilage of the Glands is often very differently affected from the viscid and saline Particles of the Blood; sometimes these Particles are mixed in different Quantities with the Mucilage, neither have the Salts at all Times the same Degree of Volatility or Fixity; so that the Mucilage may at some Times be only lightly infected, and the Infection be more Volatile, and consequently it may easily move from one Joint to another, or attack many Joints at a Time. The Points of the Salts are in a Manner lixiviated, become more volatilized, and of Consequence are with more ease protruded from the Blood into the Glands, and render the mucilaginous Juices sharper; whence the nervous Membranes are irritated and distended, and the gouty Pain generated.

SECT. 7.

The Reason why this morbid Matter is not long fixed in a Place, but is apt to wander from one Joint to another, I take to be this: These saline volatile Particles, when their intestine Motions are increased, are very easily dissipated, either through the Pores of the Skin in sensible Transpiration and Sweat, or by insensible Perspiration, and so the Pain ceases; other Glands, whose Pores are more open to receive this acrid volatile Matter, are for the like Reasons infected, the same Tragedy repeated, and the Particles in like manner dissipated. This is the Reason why the Pains in the Gout are not fixed and permanent, but rather wandring and uncertain, the morbid Particles being attenuated, and pushing to get forth by the Methods now mentioned, vellicate the Nerves in various Directions. It may be further considered, that when by the smallness of the Pores or glandulous Vessels, or any other Disposition, the morbifick Matter cannot be separated from them in sufficient Quantity, and the Secretion once begun is stopped, it recurs to other Glands of the same kind, and thus the morbid Matter is suddenly translated from one Joint to another, and from one Sett of Glands to others, so as to produce this Effect.

SECT. 8.

As to the fixed Gout, where the morbid Matter remains long in a Place, I take it that many acid Salts and viscid Humours contained in the Blood, occasion a greater Coagulation and Viscidity in the Mucilage about the Joints and the Tendons, than can be easily dispersed and evacuated; and on the contrary growing more viscid and sharp, it distends and vellicates the small Fibres of the Tendons and nervous Membranes, and occasions a Pain proportional to the Degree of Acrimony and Viscidity in the Mucilage about the Joints and Tendons, generally pretty sharp. The Mucilage is affected in the same Manner as it would be from the Affusion of *Aqua Fortis*, Spirit of Vitriol, or any other corrosive acid or austere Substance, whence it is manifestly thickned and coagulated. This affords a Reason why such a Gout is not only fixed in a particular Limb, but also why it long remains there. The ingenious Dr. *Havers* explains this Matter very well; he tells us that when the Matter happens to be thick and gelatinous, it is not to be expected that it should be easily and presently discharged out of the Interstices of the Joints, either by being resorbed or evaporated, when the Consistence of it renders it uncapable of insinuating itself into the minute Pores, and penetrating those narrow Avenues through which it is to pass. And according to the Degree and Nature of the Acid in the morbific Humour, it doth more or less coagulate the Mucilage, and the Part affected is sooner or later, with more or less Difficulty, freed from it, either by the Translation of it to another, or by the more happy Exclusion of it out of the Body. The same Author very elegantly explains the Cause of the Knots in the Joints, where he says that it seems to be no difficult Thing to account for that tophaceous Matter, which is sometimes found concreted in those Parts that have been afflicted with this Distemper. It hath been observed, that an Acid and an Austere, being both mixed with the Mucilage, did produce a plain, a notable and white Coagulation, where the *Coagulum*, though it was made when the Mucilage was cold, was not so soft and tender, nor dissolvable in Water like that which was made with Acids only; but though it would break, remained distinct in it, and being dried, was easily reducible to a fine Powder like Flower, or the fine Powder of Chalk. Whence he humbly conceives, that where-ever the Gout comes to be nodose, there is not only an Acidity in the preternatural Humour, which is separated by the mucilaginous Glands, and mixed with the Mucilage; but it is an Acid austere, which is no sooner thrown into the Interstices of the Joints and the Sinuses of the Tendons which are thereabout, but it produces a *Coagulum* in the Mucilage, and that such a one as is not easily attenuated and dissolved, so that it lies fixed and imprisoned there, and in Time, as the aqueous and moist Particles are by the Heat and Spirits carried off, the terrestrial and saline Parts concentrated come nearer together, and coming to be immediately contiguous, do mutually adhere, and are concreted so as to produce that Chalk or tophaceous Matter which is in some arthritick Cases to be observed. And as the *Coagulum*, which may be made by an Acid austere, seems apt to make a Concretion of that nature, so the Colour of the tophaceous Matter doth answer to that of this Coagulation, so as to seem generated in this Manner.

SECT. 9.

The same Author explains the Reason why the Hands and Feet are most subject to this Disorder. In the Hands, as was shewn before, there not only are considerable Glands in all their Joints, but the Tendons which are there inserted, especially those of the *Musculi perforantes*, have their mucilaginous Glands, so that Nature hath a convenience in these Parts to depurate the Mass of Blood, and they must receive the morbifick Matter, when the Blood in its Circulation obtrudes it upon them, and the Glands are disposed to separate it. The same Thing may be observed of the Shoulder and of the Knees. But of all the Parts none are so frequently afflicted with this Disease as the Feet, and it is plain why they are so. For besides, that they have many mucilaginous Glands in their Joints, and others about the Tendons which are inserted into their Bones, as the great Chord or Tendon of the Muscles which extend the Foot, and those of the *Perforantes*; I say besides this, they are the inferior and pendulous Parts, so that as their Glands make them capable of entertaining, so their Situation does conspire with the Effort of Nature, to bring down the morbifick Matter into them. Thus far Dr. *Havers*, whom I have chosen to quote, because he hath exceeded all Authors in treating of the Nature of this Distemper. It is not necessary to add any more upon this Head. What I have omitted for Brevity's Sake, the Reader may find in my *Encyclopædia Medica*, where I have treated of the Cause of this Distemper, and evidently shewed how from the Glands and Lymphatick Ducts about the Membranes and nervous Parts of the Joints, a large Quantity of sharp *Serum* and other lixivial and acid Particles or other morbid Matter thickning and corrupting the Lymph, is secreted and deposited upon the Joints, where they corrode and vellicate the nervous Fibres. Upon the Addition of Particles more than ordinary acid, the Pains become more durable and fixed; insomuch as Salts of different Natures become jumbled together, and from the Agitation and Conflict of the Particles, the Membranes are vellicated and distended in a very painful Manner; neither doth the Pain abate till the Particles get forth of the Glands, or their Conflict being over, leave the Spirits at rest.

CHAP. V.

In the next Place we are to enquire into the Properties of Milk, and to find out whence it hath such wonderful Powers in asswaging and curing this Distemper. There are some Authors, especially the Followers of *Sylvius*, who according to the chymical Scheme would have Milk produced from the Blood in the following Manner; Chyle, which is of a white Colour, may be turned into Blood by the Help of Alcalies; and again the Blood may be reduced to Chyle by the Help of Acids. *Junkius*, in his Chymistry, hath noted the Experiments when Milk is to be turned into Blood: Take a Pound of new Milk, and mix with it an Ounce of reverberated Salt of Tartar in a large Vessel; in a Quarter of an Hour the Mixture shall turn into a Blood red Colour, several Fibres swimming at Top like Cream. When the Blood is to be turned into Milk, take any Quantity of the foregoing Mixture, and drop in some Vinegar, and it shall immediately re-assume the Form of Milk. In the first Experiment they alledge, that the crude Sulphur of the Chyle is by the Alkali exalted into a red Sulphur; in the second, the exalting Alkali is depressed by the Acid, whence the Sulphur returns to its original white Colour. *Junkius* is very justly doubtful of the Application of this Experiment; how the crude Sulphur of the Chyle, as they call it, should in so short a Time be changed into Blood by Alkalies, and the Blood, exalted by so many Circulations, be again changed into Milk by Acids, seems very strange. It requires a good deal of Time to change the Chyle into perfect Blood, and the Blood again into Milk, notwithstanding that Women who have no Milk find it in their Breasts soon after Childbirth.

SECT. 2.

In order to be fully satisfied of the Nature of Milk, it is necessary to examine into the Manner of its Generation: It seems reasonable to imagine, that the Chyle, once received into the lacteal Vessels, and at length mixed with the Blood, is never again let forth with the same Appearance; only in Women at the Time of Childbirth, when it is plentifully separated, through the Ramifications of the Arteries, by the conglomerate Glands of the Breast. There is evidently a great Agreement between the Milk and the Chyle, in as much as the Chyle consists of a watry, limpid and gelatinous Fluid, with oily or fat Globules swimming therein. These Globules are pellucid, and differ both in Size and Figure; the Reason of its Whiteness is to be imputed to this: The oily Globules are mixed with the watry ones, in such Manner that several very smooth Globules are formed, which reflecting the Rays of Light in right Lines, occasion a white Colour; the same thing is observable in making Emulsions with oily Seeds, or upon mixing resinous Essences with Water, or mixing Oyl and Water, and shaking them well together; in these Cases, the watry and oily Particles, being thoroughly mixed, occasion such a Superficies as reflects a white Colour. *Bolin*, and several Authors have proved, that the Milk is no other than oily or fat Lymph or Chyle, brought with the Blood to the Breasts, and there deposited in the milky Cells. *Berger* hath very well explained the Manner of its Separation in the Breasts. The whole Substance of the Breasts, in Women giving Suck, is made up of various Ramifications of Arteries, from the thoracick and mamillary Arteries, which terminate in oval Cells, or glandulary Follicles; from hence the Breast swells with many milky Vessels, terminating in the Nipple; through these the more oily and chylous Parts of the Blood are derived from the Glands, where it is not only separated, and received, but gathered and preserved, while the remaining Mass of the Blood is returned by the Veins and Lymphaticks. These milky Rivulets, after breaking very small from the Ramifications of the Arteries, flow together into several larger Trunks, which in their Progress are united by Insertions of their Parts, in some Places more dilated, in others streightned, from several Cells and Cisterns, where the Milk is gathered and preserved, so as always to have a sufficient Quantity for the Nourishment of the Infant. Lastly, as the Chyle is separated from the Mass of the Food in the Bowels, not by any Precipitation, but by Percolation only; and as in the making of Emulsions, the oily Seeds communicate an oily Milkiness to the Water, and is separated from the grosser Parts by the Sieve, without the Intervention of any precipitating Medicine, so the chylous Juice is separated in the Bowels by gentle Pressure or the Peristaltick Motion, and strained through the Orifices of the lacteal Vessels, to be thence thrown into the Mass of the Blood. In like manner, the Milk is barely separated, by straining the milky Particles from the Blood, through the small Ramifications of the Arteries in the Glands of the Breasts.

SECT. 3.

Nuck hath sometime ago demonstrated, that these conglomerate Glands are a Bundle of small Vessels; that their excretory Ducts are Continuations of the arterial Ramifications, and that these Glands owe their Origin to the smallest Branches of the Arteries: These Arteries, which enter the glandular Substance of the Breasts, are imperceptible to the naked Eye, and discoverable only by injecting a very fine Tincture (which *Nuck* tells us is known to very few Anatomists) into the Artery; this may be so far propelled, as to render the milky Ducts conspicuous. For the better Discovery of this Matter, *Nuck* instituted another Experiment equally curious and useful; having met a Nipple full of excretory Ducts, he pressed it, and the Breast adjoining, so as to empty all its Contents, and having pitched upon one of the widest Ducts, he injected *Mercury* so artificially, that he immediately observed the milky Ducts spread like Branchings of Trees; some Part of the *Mercury* was carried so far as to enter the Arteries, whence the milky Vessels were continued.

SECT. 4.

Hence it follows, that these milky Ducts are destitute of Valves, otherwise the *Mercury* and the injected Liquors would have been obstructed in their Passage. It is indeed observable, that these Canals are in some Places streighter and narrower than in others, so as to give some kind of Obstacle to the Injection; this is not to be imputed to Valves, but to some kind of Hardness peculiar to the Substance of the Glands, by which the milky Vessels are compressed. From hence appears the immediate Inosculation of the milky Ducts, with the small Ramifications of the Arteries, of which these Glands are composed; so that the arterial Blood propels and deposits its chylous and serous Particles by gentle Pressure and Impulse in the milky Ducts, without other Mechanism than bare Straining and Secretion. For the further and more exact Description of these Ducts, see *Nuck's Adenographia.*

SECT. 5.

It remains now to examine, of what kind of Particles chiefly Milk is composed; which appear to be these three: The first is a fat, butyraceous, oily, and sulphureous Substance. The second is cheesy, earthy, chalky, and saline. The third is the Vehicle of these, *viz.* serous, which is watry, with a Mixture of nitrous Salts. But these Parts don't hold the same Proportion in the Milk of all Animals; Cows Milk is most used in Food, it is thick and fat, and contains more Butter than the Milk of other Animals; upon which account it nourishes more, and is more agreeable to the human Body. Ews Milk hath more earthy and cheesy Particles; Goats Milk is in a Mean between these two, only that its *Serum* contains more of a nitrous Salt; whence *Etmuller* conjectures, that it hath all the Virtues of Whey made from Cows Milk, especially in Heats and scorbutick Cases. Asses Milk is of all the thinnest, next to human; the Milk of other Animals, as not so usually brought into Food, I forbear to describe.

SECT. 6.

It is manifest, that every Part of the Milk exerts an Effect proper to it self; the fat Part, from which the Butter is formed, preserves from the Stone, which affords an evident Reason why Stones taken from the human Body, upon Distillation, afford so small a Portion of Oyl; whence I am of Opinion, that the Stone is most commonly generated in the Kidneys and

Bladder, when the Blood is not sufficiently stocked with oily Particles. Upon this Principle it is easy to see why all oily Substances, as Oyl of Sweet Almonds, taken plentifully, is a Remedy in the Stone; for the oily Particles (as *Hoffman* observes in his Notes upon *Poterius*) by their Hooks hinder the Saline *Spicula* from uniting so as to form an hard Substance. It is known in the Chymistry, that Oyl resists Crystallization; and many Artists that are minded to have beautiful Crystals, add rectified Spirit of Wine to their Lye, in order to absorb the Oyl. Upon the same Principles, the Precipitation of the earthy Particles, and the lodging thereof in the Membranes of the Joints, so as to form chalky Knots, are prevented. *Poterius* tells us of a Woman of Sixty, who was so reduced in her Flesh and Strength, that she was scarce sensible of Pain, who by the Help of Goat's Milk, was in three Months Time restored to a State of perfect Health, notwithstanding a great Decay of Strength and Flesh, an Hectick Fever, and a Stone; she took at first but four Ounces of the Milk, which was at length increased to eight; at the End of fifteen Days she voided some oblong and Very hard Stones, upon which she began to recover. She continued the Use of the Milk for a Month, at which Time the Fever left her, her Appetite returned, and she began to gather Flesh. She was alive and hearty in the Sixty Eighth Year of her Age, when *Poterius* gave his Account. Although in this Case the oily Particles of the Blood might contribute much to lubricate the Passages, yet probably the serous Part of the Goats Milk, impregnated with a nitrous abstersive Salt, attenuated the thicker Humours, and irritated the nervous membranous Parts to discharge the Stones. It is observable that after taking plentifully of Milk, the Urine is not only thin and watry, but made also in large Quantities. This fat Substance in the Milk also loosens the Bowels and softens Pain, it resists corrosive Poisons, in as much as it sheaths and anoints the sharp *Spicula* thereof. Many Empiricks, to shew the Force of their Antidotes (which are generally good for nothing) to the ignorant Multitude, having lined their Stomachs well with Butter, or Oyl, either of Olive or Sweet Almonds, will securely swallow Mercury and even Arsenick, and afterwards taking the pretended Specifick, cheat the poor People of their Money. *Poterius* experienced the good Effects of Milk, plentifully taken, to break the Force of Poyson; for a Woman, who being very dry, had drank *Aqua Fortis* instead of Wine, was relieved from the immediate Danger of Death by drinking plentifully of Steeled Milk, with a Dram of Wax, a little Nutmeg, and *Terra Lemnia*. *Tulpius*, in his Observations takes Notice, that *Goldsmiths*, while they handle Mercury and Antimony, keep in their Mouths a bit of Bread thick buttered, or take fat Broths, to guard against their mischievous *Effluvia*. Milk, by reason of its Oiliness, is one of the best, temperate, and nourishing of Foods; nothing exceeds it in consumptive Cases. These Particles admirably temper any Sharpness in the Body, and are serviceable where the Kidneys are ulcerated, and to scorbutick People, especially if the Juice of Cresses or Scurvygrass be added to it, and taken two Hours before Meals. It is of great Service in Dysenteries, where there is great Sharpness in the first Passages, and chiefly after the Use of absorbent Medicines. Upon the same Account it eases Pains in the Eyes, and the serous Part of the Milk helps much to dilute the Salts; dropt into the Ear, it asswages Pains there, especially when it is attended with a buzzing Noise.

SECT. 7.

Since it appears that Milk, by reason of its oily Particles, is thus serviceable in mitigating and curing these Disorders, there is no room to doubt, from Parity of Reason, that the frequent Use of it in the Gout should not break and invert the austere, sharp, saline Particles, and drive them forth of the Body by Perspiration, Urine, or other Discharges; for, (as *Waldsmid* observes) Salts predominate in this Distemper, which is evident from the itching in the Skin observed to attend the Decline of a Fit. The volatile Salt of the serous Humour going off, insensibly frets the Skin, while that which is fixed in the thick and viscid Humour, and cannot easily fly off, hardens into Knots. I have observed, upon the Application of Blisters to gouty Persons, a Liquor of an high corrosive Nature to flow from the Part.

SECT. 8.

I now come to examine the second essential Part of Milk, *viz.* that which is cheesy, earthy, and somewhat saline. I am not of Opinion that the Acid of the Stomach is increased by this Part, for there is no Acid naturally in the Stomach; if there were, it would be mischievous. Although it be certain that Cheese is acid, and turns sharper by Age, yet those Particles which are precipitated into Chese, are vastly different in the Chyle and the Milk, from what they are in a State of Separation, and after being exposed to the Air. The Salts, which before were nitrous, and of a middle Nature, somewhat volatile, and mixed with oily, sulphureous, or earthy Particles, being agitated by an inward Motion, become more stiff and complicated. These Salts, while in a State of Union with the Milk and Chyle in the Body, by Means of the progressive Motion, are more disunited and smaller, the serous and oily Particles keeping them asunder; and there is neither Time nor Rest allowed them in their natural State to produce fresh Combinations, as they have when deprived of their progressive Motion, in a State of Separation from the Body. That Milk in warm Weather turns sowre, is to be imputed to its intestine Motion, where the Salts, before small and somewhat nitrous, mixed with the oily Particles by the Influx of the Air, change their natural Texture and Figure, and become more rigid and heavy, and so precipitate the light, viscid, and earthy Particles. That the Air contributes much to this

Change, appears from hence, because that alone produces a remarkable Quantity of acid Salts in some Bodies. If a Piece of Alum be calcined in the open Fire, upon exposing it again to the Air, it shall double its Weight; so that a large Quantity of aluminous acid Salt may be drawn from thence: And although Milk be coagulated in the Breasts, it happens either from an acid Acrimony in the Blood, or its Motion being stopped, and some Obstructions of the milky Vessels. It doth not appear from any Experiment yet known, that healthy Milk fresh drawn contains any Acid; the Manner in which this Part of the Milk acquires this Tendency, I conceive to be this: We have already asserted, that Milk, in its natural State, contains no Acid, although after being exposed to Warm Air, by Means of some Fermentation and inward Motion, it becomes acid, which is to be look'd upon as a new Production, no way relating to Milk in its natural State. The cheesy Particles of Milk, if I may so call them, when in the Body differ extremely from those which out of the Body form the Cheese; for while in the Body, they are in the Shape of earthy, subtile, viscid Particles, mixed with the Milk, Chyle, and Blood; they give a due Consistence to the Milk, by duly mixing the oily, fat and serous Particles with them, and while in their due progressive Motion, keep the Milk in a proper Temperature, and occasion a slower Motion of the Milk through the milky Vessels.

SECT. 9.

It may be asked, How this Part of the Milk comes to be serviceable in the Gout, and other scorbutick Disorders? Because its Parts are slimy, chalky, and earthy, they gently temper the Acrimony of the Humours, and imbibe and absorb it; and this is the Reason why the Milk of Nurses who feed upon Acids, or whose Blood hath a Tendency that Way, soon turns; for such acid Particles being separated in the Glands of the Breasts, by coagulating and thinning the Milk, by separating from the other Particles of the Milk, and staying behind, are the Occasion that the Milk comes out unfit for Nourishment.

SECT. 10.

The third Part of the Milk, which is serous, contains watry, gelatinous and nitrous Particles; if Milk sowres and coagulates out of the Body, the gelatinous Parts of the *Serum*, being somewhat thicker and more earthy, change their Motion and Situation, and being more closely mixed with the oily Particles, become that cheesy Substance we before took Notice of. The Power of the *Serum* is to be attributed to its watry and abstersive nitrous Particles, by Means whereof it hath a Power of deterging, consolidating, sweetning and tempering the Acrimony of the Humours, and of increasing the Discharges by Urine and Siege; it removes Obstructions in the Bowels, heals Ulcers, and corrects the Sharpness of the Humours, in as much as it dilutes the acrid and volatile Salts, and fixes them by means of its nitrous Particles. It is of great use in feverish Heats, and by its alexipharmick Power is much esteemed in malignant Fevers, so that its Virtue in the Gout is less to be wondered at. In the Gout, the fixed morbid Matter sticking in the small Canals, and the Interstices of the Membranes and mucilaginous Glands, is very tough, viscid, sharp and austere; the serous Particles of the Milk easily pass through and pervade those Ducts and Canals, and by the watry Particles dilute those sharp Salts and stagnating Humours, and partly imbibe and absorb them; so that either by insensible Perspiration, Urine, or some other Discharge, they send them forth of the Body. For this End they correct and break them so as to make their Passage easier. It is observable, that the Salts of the *Serum* easily assimilate themselves to other Salts, and upon this Account a difference of Food occasions different Milk. Goats that have fed upon purging Herbs, Spurge or Scammony, as in *Syria* or other Countries where such Herbs grow wild, give Milk endowed with a strong purgative Power; and Saffron frequently given communicates both its Smell and Colour to the Milk.

SECT. 11.

For these Reasons those that feed upon Milk should take Care that the Animal they take it from have sweet and good Pasture; Cows give sweeter and better Milk in Summer, when fed upon odoriferous Grass, than in Winter on Hay and Straw. I do not think it necessary here, to recite all the Virtues of the serous Part of the Milk in the Cure of other Distempers, because they are well known to Physicians; but it may be observed, that the several essential Parts of Milk, which I have here explained, being united and thoroughly mixed, as they are in the Milk, exert a greater Efficacy in dissolving and breaking the Salts and viscid Humours that lodge about the Joints, and expelling the gouty Matter. When the Blood is impregnated with Milk, it yields a softer Liquor to the mucilaginous Glands of the Joints, so that the Membranes and Tendons are lubricated with a soft insipid Mucilage, and the natural Motions are performed without Pain or Uneasiness; or if the Membranes be too dry, or complicated with any sharp Matter, which occasions Obstructions, they are so relaxed, that upon removing the Obstruction they regain their former Force and Vigour. Care must be taken of what I before advised, that before the Milk be thoroughly brought into Use, the latent Acid in the Bowels be first corrected and discharged by absorbent and cleansing Medicines, and a laudable Diet premised for some Time, that no Coagulation of the Milk, or other Inconveniencies, be incurred. Upon this Foot a certain Cure is to be expected. A prudent Physician will easily dispose a Body whose Powers are not entirely destroyed to receive this Diet. Perhaps some may object here, that the Gout being caused by an acid Salt, rendring the Juices about the

Joints more viscid and sharp, therefore so long as there remains a Disposition to the Gout, from this Cause, Milk cannot safely be brought into Use. To this I answer, That the Gout is often caused by a singular lixivial Salt, and bilious Acrimony, especially in Persons of a sanguine Constitution, where no volatile Acid is observable, either in the first Passages, or in the Blood; or if there be any acid Salts in the first Passages, by frequent Circulations they are so joined with the volatile Salt of the Blood, that they become lixivial and bilious. But when there really are acid Humours in the Body, by taking alcaline Absorbents and Cleansers of the Blood, and by proper Diet, they may be so corrected, as from Acids to become lixivial, and assume the Nature of middle Kind of Salts. Upon the frequent Use of alkaline Absorbents, the Pains of the Gout are mightily lessened, because the solid *Spicula* of the Acid are broke and changed. Upon this Principle, Dr. *Willis* his Mixture of the Solution of Salt of Tartar, and *Sal Ammoniac*, in Rain Water, externally applied, is an excellent Remedy. A Friend of mine used to remove the Pains of the Gout instantly, by an Ointment made of Quick Lime; and upon the same Principles, Spirit of *Sal Ammoniac*, Camphire, Spirit and Oyl of Tartar, and even Urine, wonderfully remove the Pain; as also Spirit of Scurvygrass, Cresses, *Sal Volatile*, Amber, and others of that Class. When the Humours that cause the Gout are more bilious, lixivial, and corrosive, these Medicines are not so proper; for volatile and spirituous Medicines increase the Distemper; but the more fixed nitrous Absorbents, oily and acid, ought to be externally applied; as Balsam of *Sulphur* with Amber, Bathing, and Spirit of Pismires, sowre Buttermilk, Herring Brine, the Juice of Earthworms expressed with Wine, as being full of nitrous Salts, a Poultice of Bread and Milk, with a little Saffron, or Bole, or sealed Earth, or the inward Use of the Decoctions of the Woods, and many other earthy Absorbents. *Caspar Rheinbold,* his Highness's Principal Apothecary, prepares a Medicine from Gold chemically, which is an admirable Secret in the Cure of the Gout, of which I can attest the Truth. It is also excellent in the Stone, prevents its growing, and mitigates the Pain of it. The Antients exhibited the Juice of Earthworms expressed in Milk, with Success: By these Means the corrosive and volatile Salts are inverted, fixed, and thrown forth of the Body by Urine and Sweat.

SECT. 12.

Because the morbid Matter rests chiefly about the Tendons and nervous Membranes, especially in the mucilaginous Glands, and cannot suddenly and at one Push be driven out of such narrow Vessels and Cells; it is necessary to continue the Diet for a good while, till the Body be thoroughly purged of vicious Humours, and begins as it were to renew its Youth.

Lenient and laxative Purgers are sometimes to be used, because the Stomach and Bowels in gouty Persons are weak; so that it often happens that Milk, by reason of the slow Progress of Chylification, by its intestine Motion, is vehemently agitated and precipitated, so as to occasion a Slime in the first Passages; but in a little Time this Evil is prevented by such Medicines as strengthen the Stomach, and prevent Coagulations in the Milk; the most lenient Purgatives are the best, and Rhubarb to be preferred for at the same Time that it evacuates, it gives a fresh Tone to the Fibres of the Bowels.

SECT. 13.

The Excellency of Milk, not only in the Gout, but in other Disorders, having been thus demonstrated, I shall subjoin the Judgment of some Authors in its Favour. *Emmanuel Konig*, in his *Regnum Animale*, admires the wonderful Power of Milk in Medicine, as well as Nourishment. *Wepfer*, in his Observations, says, there is certainly somewhat divine in Milk, since we see gouty Persons relieved by it, Hypocondriack and Nephritick Persons relieved by its use, the whole Habit strengthened, the Complexion cleared up, and fresh Powers acquired to the Body. He tells us, that he knew a Gentlewoman at *Friburgh*, who was in an almost miraculous Manner relieved from terrible Convulsions, Suffocation of the Womb, Hysterick Symptoms, by the Use of Milk alone, obstinately persisted in for some Years. Milk, by its asswaging, sulphureous Power, and its nitro-saline deterging Quality, dulcifies the sharp and acid Humours, whence its Cream and Butter thence arising, are very anodine; the one beat up with Sugar of Lead, corrects the corrosive Acid in cancerous Tumours; and the other drank warm in a *Diarrhœa*, mitigates the sharp Twitches in the Bowels that attend that Distemper, and immediately asswages and stops the Pain and Gripings. Externally applied and rubbed in a proper manner, it gives Relief in the Stone, and helps to propel it into the Bladder. *Daniel Ludovicus* hath asserted, that Butter either by it self, or mixed with other Ingredients, exceeds all the Officinal Ointments and compound Oyls. In Consumptions and Hecticks its Powers are very well known. *Solenander* and *Konig* advise a Pound of Milk, in which an Handful of Elder Flowers have been boiled, drank every Morning for nine Days successively in *May*, as a Specifick in St. *Anthony*'s Fire. *Tachius* tells us of what great Use it was in restoring crippled Limbs to a Person that was quite tired out with Baths, and other Remedies. In the *German Ephemeris* there is an Instance of an Hypocondriac Epilepsy cured by three Ounces of Milk, in which was dissolved half a Drachm of *Spanish* Soap, taken every Morning. And *Sylvius* tells us of many Icterical People cured by that Medicine.

CHAPTER. VI.

Before I finish this Discourse, I shall endeavour to give some Account why People that have been cured by this Method, and have lived many Years free from the Gout, at certain Times of the Year, particularly upon Change of Weather, or at that Time of the Year when they used to have the Fits, perceive some slight and obscure Pains about the Joints of those Limbs that were formerly attacked. This I suppose to arise from the Blood and Humours being thickned by the preternatural Influence of the Air at those Seasons; if upon such a Cause the Humours become thicker in the mucilaginous Glands, the Membranes must of course be distended. Now because this doth not proceed from any particular Acrimony, but from a Fullness and slight Distention, therefore the Pain thence arising is hardly perceivable, and vanishes upon gentle Exercise and walking, in which the Motion of the Blood is a little increased.

SECT. 2.

It is necessary in the next Place to propose and confute some Objections of Persons who refuse this Diet as extremely noxious. Altho', *say they*, Persons have found great Benefit by strictly adhering to this Diet, yet upon returning again to the Use of common Food, however mild and gentle, they have been afflicted with the Gout worse than ever. The Powers of the Body being weakned by this Diet, have been less able to resist the Force of this Distemper, it hath become more dangerous, and the Fits of longer Continuance. If we may give Credit to Experience as well as Reason, we shall find this Matter far otherwise, for it appears from what we have said, that many Persons have not only been freed from the Gout in this Method, but have likewise continued free many Years after they have left it off; particularly the three Gentlemen now living at the *Hague*, the Marquiss *de Bongi*, Monsieur *Chamar*, and the Counsellour *de Talo*. It is observable, that having gone through the Diet, they returned to different kinds of Food, and have now lived with their Friends as usual without any Inconvenience for several Years, excepting the Marquiss, who twice or thrice in the Compass of nine or ten Years hath been afflicted with it, (probably owing to some Error in the Non-Naturals;) it is no less reasonable to believe, that where the Aliments are easier changed into good Chyle, and communicated to the Blood in proper Quantities, better Spirits should be produced, and of Consequence the Vigour of the Parts should be restored and augmented. That this is natural to Milk, appears from common Experience in the Diet of such as use chiefly Milk and Water, (as the Country People in *Switzerland*) for they exceed those of other Countries and Places who live upon Flesh-

Meats, in the Largeness and Health of their Bodies, and the Floridness of their Complections, and you shall seldom find any among them subject to the Gout, the Scurvy, Hypochondriack, or other Distempers.

SECT. 3.

If any object that gouty Persons, in the Beginning of the Diet, find their Stomach and Limbs weakned by the Milk, so that they have need of Stomachick and other strengthening Medicines, let it be remembred that the Glands of the Stomach and Bowels in gouty Persons, that furnish the Stomachick and intestinal Juices, are obstructed and furred with a viscid kind of Matter, so that only the more subtile and liquid Fluids can enter their Pores; hence the watry Part of the Milk, with very few oily nutritious Particles, enter those Pores and Canals, so that the Chyle becomes too watry, not being sufficiently impregnated with a proper Quantity of oily Particles. This Chyle not being sufficiently stored with nutritious Particles, being delivered into the Blood, occasions a Languor and Weakness, while the thicker Parts of the Milk go off with the Excrement. But after a while, when the watry Parts of the Milk have frequently entered the Mass of the Blood, and have resolved, imbibed and inverted the corrosive Salts that coagulate the Humours, and expelled them by Perspiration or Urine; then by Degrees, those Humours that are separated in the Glands, and serve to the Concoction and Digestion of the Aliment, as the Spittle, the Juices of the Stomach and Bowels, the Bile, the pancreatick Juice, become thinner, and the Canals and Pores of those Glands are rendred fit, not only to receive the watry Parts of the Milk, but the oily nutritious Parts also, and of forming them into good and laudable Chyle. The Reason why gouty People using their ordinary Aliment, retain more Strength and Vigour, is this, not only the Pores of the Glands of the Stomach and Bowels are by long use more apt to admit Particles from their ordinary Food, but its Parts also are more thick and heavy, so that the chylous Part is protruded by the Weight of the superincumbent Particles. To this concurrs a particular Acrimony, by Means whereof the Coats of the Stomach are vellicated, and exert a greater Force in separating the Chyle, whereas Milk which presses more gently, does not so easily enter Pores stuffed with viscid Humours, but rather insinuates itself by Degrees in those Canals where it can find Passage. If the Tone of the Bowels be in a natural State, and the first Passages be not loaded with acid and viscid Humours, Milk from a natural Affinity, is more easily converted into Chyle, and nourishes and strengthens the Body more than any other Food, which takes more Time in its Digestion, especially if some fine unfermented Wheaten Bread be taken along with it; for by this Means the Parts of the Chyle are rendred more heavy, and easily enter the lacteal Vessels, communicate a solid Nourishment to the Body, and the

Strength thereof is mightily restored, without the least Hazard of any Damage.

SECT. 4.

Notwithstanding what I have endeavoured to prove, that gouty Persons, after having been cured by this Method, may again return to their common way of living, without fear of a Relapse; yet I do not deny but it is an easy matter to bring on the Gout again, and that in a more violent Manner than before, by great Errors in Diet, indulging in acid Foods, smoaked Meats, and such as are flatulent and of bad Digestion; too frequent drinking of acid and generous Wines; giving way to the Passions of Anger and Sorrow, the use of Women, or being exposed to the Inclemencies of the Air. No doubt these will return the Distemper with great Violence, and bring the Patient into manifest danger. It is absolutely necessary to chuse such Food as will give Chyle analogous to Milk, and to avoid all Acid and Salt Food with the greatest Caution. And although some People have indulged their Appetites after the Cure, without any great Inconvenience, yet it is certainly more advisable to live moderately, since too much Boldness is not always successful; which the Patient will certainly be encouraged to do, upon recalling to mind the terrible Pains he hath suffered, hardly relievable by any Art.

SECT. 5.

It may be enquired how it comes to pass, that a Person cured by this Diet shall continue free from the Gout, though he return to his former Method of living, provided he take every Morning a small Quantity of warm Milk. The Reason of this I take to be, that the Milk, by long Use, during the Time of the Cure, hath either changed or expelled all the sharp Acrimony of the Blood and Humours, and rendred the Fibres and Membranes more loose, so that there is an easier Circulation of the Juices; new acid Salts are not so easily formed and thrown upon the Membranes so as to occasion the Gout, especially if the Diet be of a good Kind, and a certain Quantity of Milk taken every Morning, which by its plentiful oily Parts, and soft serous ones, prevents the Salts from uniting. I am sensible I may have omitted some Doubts that might arise against the Use of this Diet, but whatever they be, they may easily be answered from what was said before, and the Use thereof fully cleared up; for lesser Difficulties, it is not worth while to spend Time about them. I shall only add, that several People have expected the Cure of the Gout in the Use of Gruels and Water. As to Water, it is evident from Experience, as *Poterius* and *Hoffman* have observed, that it is frequently serviceable in removing this Distemper. Since gouty Persons are of a saline Constitution, there cannot be a better drink used than pure light Water, that will make its way both by the Skin and by Urine;

for such drank freely drives forth the foreign Salts, and makes the Juices fluid. I have seen Persons cured of the Gout, whose Joints were contracting, by drinking only pure Spring Water in large Quantities. The Case of a Man, who was a Cripple for nine Years successively, from an ill cured Tertian, deserves Observation. He drank of the Water of this Place, which is very wholesome and something Vitriolick, for a Month together, sometimes to the Quantity of eight Quarts; he made Urine plentifully, and came gradually to the Use of his Hands and Feet; so that he could both walk and gripe any thing with his Hands in a short Time, to the Admiration of all those who knew his Condition before. From hence it appears, that large Quantities of Water do no Mischief, but by the Pressure are most powerfully deobstruent. I knew a gouty Gentleman who drank warm Beer with great Success in the Gout; and the *Chinese*, who drink their Water warm, are not subject to this Distemper. There are various Ways of removing Obstructions, and tempering the Acrimony of the Juices, but we are very much in doubt, whether by these Methods the very Cause of the Gout can be so thoroughly extirpated and conveniently cured, as by the Use of Milk; for Water drank in too great Quantities (as it is not endowed with any nutritious Particles) weakens the Tone of the Bowels, and damps the vital heat; though if it be used with Caution, in Distempers arising from an Acrimony of the Juices, it is very often of great Efficacy.

CPSIA information can be obtained
at www.ICGtesting.com
Printed in the USA
BVHW032343251021
619846BV00007B/567